PASTORAL CARE IN HEALTH FACILITIES

A Book of Readings

Edited by

Ward A. Knights, Jr.
Supervisor of Clinical Pastoral Education
Saint Joseph's Hospital
Saint Paul, Minnesota

THE CATHOLIC HOSPITAL ASSOCIATION
St. Louis, Missouri 63104

Copyright © 1977
by
The Catholic Hospital Association
St. Louis, Missouri 63104

Printed in the U.S. of America. All
rights reserved. This book, or any
part thereof, may not be reproduced
without the written permission of the
publisher.

Library of Congress Catalog Card No. 76-26994

ISBN 0-87125-035-7

To
Ellen and Laura
and
Hazel
and
Elaine and Laura

TREASURES TO BE FOUND

Adventurous healers,
Risking submersion in the hidden, dark depths
  of people in pain,
  Enduring the inevitable entanglements in webs
  woven of sickness, fear and dread.
Why risk these hazards?
  Because there are *treasures to be found.*
How can you be so sure?
  Because you have one buried within yourself.
You have awaited diagnosis.
  You have known isolation.
You have scars.

In truth then, these are not uncharted lands.
There are trails, winding but well-worn.
  Your own remembered darknesses now bring light
    into the shadows of other's sufferings.
Memory of past pain
  Is the needle on your compass.

The treasure: Compassion,
Buried in the earth of your own aches,
  In the ground enriched
In the time of desolation.

By sharing your wounds, you grow rich together.

Fortunate healers!

Wayne L. Hornicek

Preface

It was by chance, or perhaps what theologians might wish to call the Grace of God, that I became involved in the field of pastoral care and counseling. That involvement was prompted by the personal needs of others which I had the audacity to assume I could respond to as a pastor.

I learned early that the task every pastor faces is a difficult one, requiring him to be a knowledgeable and whole person. The knowledge and experience that are required are not easily come by, and the process of achieving them is never complete. Each piece of knowledge, each bit of personal growth, leads to yet more knowledge and points to yet more needed growth.

Ministering to persons experiencing illness is one of the most difficult, yet most rewarding, tasks of a pastor. Today, more than ever before, it requires special knowledge and experience. It requires the pastoral person, clergy or layman, to have a genuine appreciation of patienthood, an in-depth understanding, for example, of the uniqueness of what it means to be a cancer patient and what this means in terms of pastoral ministry.

Such understanding requires highly specialized training, one form of which is Clinical Pastoral Education. My personal pilgrimage brought me to CPE as I sought to grow and become effective in my service to others. Subsequent experiences in pastoral ministries in churches, mental hospitals, and general hospitals convinced me that pastoral ministry is enhanced when we are open to learning from one another, when there is mutual sharing on a personal and professional level.

This manuscript is an attempt to share on the part of many people most of whom are my personal friends, colleagues, or students. My sincerest appreciation goes to each one of them for their unique contribution, as well as for the personal pastoral care which many of them have given to me.

In a very real sense this manuscript represents the work of the Department of Pastoral Care at St. Joseph's Hospital and of its Director, Fr. David M. McPhee. I want to express my appreciation to Sr. Marie DePaul Rochester for her understanding and effective administrative support, both of which are making possible the conditions under which modern professional pastoral care can be practiced. My most special thanks go to Mrs. Ethel Gleason who, with diligent labor and great love, helped in the preparation of this manuscript.

The chapter titled "The Hospital Chaplain and the Patient's Family" by Fr. McPhee appeared in the October 1972 issue of *Hospital Progress*, and an edited version is being reprinted with permission of *Hospital Progress*.

This book does not presume to have touched all the specialized areas of pastoral care in illness. Rather, it attempts to give a representative presentation of pastoral care.

Ward A. Knights, Jr.

Contents

A Holistic Concept of Illness

DALE DOBSON, DD

The ultimate in patient care is the practice of "holistic" medicine. Quite simply, holistic medicine refers to care of the total patient, including anatomical, physiological, psychological, and environmental aspects. Hippocrates was the first person to advocate holistic care. This concept recognizes that the body is not merely a group of independent organs and systems, but is a complex, interrelated community of organs and systems, each dependent on the other, each contributing to the other, each compensating for the other to meet the constant demands of internal and external stress.

In diagnosing and treating patients, physicians who follow the holistic approach are guided by certain generally accepted principles concerning normal functioning of the body.

First, the human body is a unit, an integrated organism in which no part functions independently. Abnormal structure or function in one part of the body creates unfavorable changes in other areas and, therefore, involves the body as a whole. The emotional and psychological influences on illness are important considerations.

The common tendency today is to isolate illness within certain structures or systems. We must recognize that when the body is sick, it is sick all over. Although a specific organ may be the central focus of illness, the effects of the illness are felt in varying degrees throughout the body. It is also important to realize that, in responding to illness, the target organ does not work alone. The whole body mounts the attack, utilizing the circulatory, endocrine, and nervous systems to counteract the effect of the illness. Recovery is achieved only when the total body returns to its normal balance.

A second principle is that the body, utilizing its complex system of checks and balances, is self-regulating and heals itself when confronted with disease, stress, or noxious influences. Health and illness are not separate and distinct entities. Rather than rest in a state of health or illness, the body constantly fluctuates between the two. The body adapts itself to the changing demands of its environment, including internal as well as external factors. It must neutralize the continual physical and psychic stresses to which it is subjected. Our state of health is determined by how well our body and mind adapt to the stresses of life. If they do well, we will be healthy. If some adverse condition interferes with our adaptive ability and disturbs the internal equilibrium, we become ill.

For most persons, illness is an infrequent occurrence despite the constant stresses of life. This fact indicates that the body is often able to resist disease and overcome illness without us necessarily being aware of the intricate actions and reactions occurring.

Pastoral counseling has assumed increased responsibility as medical practice has been altered by intrinsic and extrinsic factors. The physician formerly served the role of physician, scientist, counselor, friend, and sounding board for his patients. However, with the increasing complexity of our world today and the physician shortage, the trend towards specialization has increased, with the physician serving a more limited and sharply defined role. The rapid growth of medical and scientific information, both technical and philosophical, has been overwhelming and has contributed to specialization and superspecialization, with the result that physicians know more and more about limited areas of the body.

Medical schools did not anticipate the population explosion and the number of physicians has not kept pace with population growth. Significant actions by federal, state, and medical authorities will correct the physician shortage, but a lag time is inevitable.

These developments encourage the team approach to holistic medical care, and the pastoral counselor is a very important member of this team. For the counselor, the most significant aspect of the holistic approach is the emotional or psychic component of disease. It is important to note that emotional and psychic components are major contributors to disease, and that decreasing these emotional factors frequently allows the body to overcome the physical and physiological stresses. Certain diseases, such as ulcers and some colitis syndromes, are closely associated with emotional stress. Less obvious but equally important are the emotional aspects of essential hypertension, cardiac problems, and many other symptoms and/or diseases.

It is said that we are products of our environment, and this is particularly true with respect to our state of health. Environmental stress is produced not only by noxious chemicals, noise, and physical stress, but also by our quest for security and happiness through interrelationships with friends, enemies, co-workers, church, government, and employers.

It is in the area of stress that the counselor can make a major contribution to total health care. Cooperation between the physician, counselors, employers, family, and government is necessary to make a holistic approach to health care possible.

Clinical Preparation for Pastoral Care and Counseling:

A Spiritual-Existential-Humanistic Approach

THE REV. WARD A. KNIGHTS, JR., D.DIV.

During the past 50 years, Clinical Pastoral Education (CPE) has evolved and grown as an accepted method of training for pastoral care and counseling. It developed because of a need for clinical experience for those working in the field of pastoral care and counseling. The idea that a person could be an adequate minister if he "read theology" and learned the appropriate rituals gradually gave way to a recognition that adequate pastoral care involved knowledge and understanding of a wider spectrum of human experience.

In the early years of CPE development, medical education was widely used as a model, and both psychology and education made their contributions. However, this approach, however much it had to offer, did not provide completely accurate or appropriate models. The pastor does not approach his people as does a physician who heals the sick, nor as one who assesses human functioning, nor as one who teaches those without information. The pastor's role, while it may encompass certain aspects of these activities, is still distinctively different. Perhaps the difference can best be indicated by saying that the pastoral approach is spiritual-existential-humanistic. Therefore, clinical preparation for pastoral care and counseling must also be unique.

THE BASIC ORIENTATION OF CPE PROGRAMS

The *first* and most basic aspect of CPE is that it is a spiritual program. There would be no need for CPE apart from the need to prepare people to meet the religious needs of others, to represent the Church. This is the foundation on which the program is built and which permeates its entire structure and content. It is motivated by service to others, and it meets the needs of people both by utilizing traditional religious resources and by searching for new, innovative forms of ministry.

Second, it acknowledges that everyone who is associated with the program is involved with fellow human beings. People are seen not as units to be diagnosed, or as data to be investigated clinically, or simply as pawns in some other-worldly chess game, but rather as fellow human beings. They are real, alive, thinking, feeling individuals in their own unique situations. They are seeking to find meaning in their lives, celebrate purpose, cope with crisis, overcome negative experiences, live with pain and suffering.

The truly professional person in pastoral care and counseling is involved with these concerns on a broad scale, and knows that the factors which bring each person to where he is are often intricate in structure. Accordingly, all attempts to help the individual must take care not to over-simplify and must reach the sources of the disturbance before significant change can occur. At the same time, the apparently simple act of listening to another person or just being with him can be a most effective form of ministry. Most important, pastoral care is for all people, not just something for a specific "faith group" or for "good church goers."

Third, CPE is existential. It is *not* basically a classroom experience. It is a full-time involvement in which the participant lives in the situation and has an in-depth experience of it. The persons and situations encountered are real, not just case histories in a textbook. In the CPE program, students encounter the vital experiences of joy, fear, frustration, pain, and death in face-to-face situations. Only in this way can would-be pastoral counselors truly gain a "feel" for these realities. Only by this type of first-hand experience can the ability and skill to minister to others be honed to a cutting edge.

The existential approach encourages the student to let his feelings and imagination run free and to set aside the limits often imposed by custom and tradition. In this way, it encourages new and creative actions. This approach also helps students set aside the false body-mind or body-soul dichotomy which has plagued pastoral care and counseling, and regain the Biblical concept of man as an holistic being. The

CPE student experiences persons, himself included, as holistic (all of one piece), and he realizes the importance of this basic fact. This approach also enables him to see more clearly the nobility and strength of human nature, which even religion has not always recognized and honored.

Fourth, while CPE stresses experience, it does not denigrate knowledge. Quite the contrary. Knowledge becomes more important to the individual in CPE because it becomes alive by being related directly to persons, to living experience. For example, while we might "know" that withdrawal is one possible reaction to stress, if we can struggle with a person, be part of the hell in which he lives because of his withdrawal, and do this in a truly empathic way, we gain a "knowledge" of withdrawal that we could achieve in no other way.

Fifth, CPE is a process of continual learning and growth — both for students and staff. Since competence is the main factor which distinguishes involvement, traditional relationships, arbitrary authority, or special privilege are quickly disposed of in CPE. While the CPE supervisor will have his own position, his own knowledge, his preferred way of doing things, the student is encouraged to seek and find the way *he* functions most effectively. Effectiveness with people is the first and foremost criterion for success in a CPE program. Effectiveness is partially determined by input from others, including the supervisor of the program, but in the last analysis, it is a judgment made by the CPE course participant. Likewise the supervisor continually changes, modifies, and refines the program in terms of what makes for the best experience for students, and, through this process, he constantly reevaluates his own pastoral theology.

Sixth, CPE respects the individuality and creativity of each student. It assumes that each person is capable of setting goals for personal involvement and of deciding how they may best be pursued. No other position is possible if the humanness of the pastoral person is truly appreciated. Of course, this position implies that the student possesses self-awareness as well as awareness of things outside himself — a true appreciation of the Gestalt of his own experience. Where such awareness is minimal, the program allows for work in this area as part of the student's individualized program. CPE provides opportunity for personal growth in recognition of the fact that only a person who is whole himself can minister to others.

Seventh, CPE recognizes *realities* rather than reality. This is sometimes a hard truth for those brought up in religious and theological traditions that did not allow for pluralism in human experience. Modern pastoral care and counseling insists that we can understand a given person only insofar as we apprehend his "internal frame of reference." No "external frame of reference" can be relevant to a person's need, without a deep understanding of how a person perceives his own experience. CPE has always stressed this very important factor. Not only psychological theory but also theology is seen in this way.

WHAT WE DO AND HOW WE DO IT

Although, in general, CPE programs have similar content, they vary widely because each is adapted to fit the particular situation in which it exists. Therefore, even programs in the same setting will vary considerably from unit to unit. Nevertheless, although techniques, approaches, and content may vary, all CPE programs expect high student achievement.

Psychoanalytic theory and technique have always occupied a respected place in CPE. The empathic, listening approach of Carl Rogers is often considered a model for pastoral sensitivity and response. Other approaches that are also used include a rational-emotive approach and a Gestalt orientation. However, no one approach is seen as the final answer to the questions that surround human experience. Rather, CPE is seen as a "smorgasbord," containing a wide variety of theories, techniques, and approaches. CPE is not a program for those who want to focus in narrowly on one approach to helping people. It is for those who are open to ever-expanding discoveries about themselves and others, and who choose an approach on the basis of a person's need rather than on the basis of a predetermined position.

CPE is offered in basic units of eleven weeks each. It takes place in a variety of settings, ranging from mental and general hospitals, to pastoral counseling centers, schools for the mentally retarded, penal and correctional institutions, juvenile treatment centers, parishes and intercity ministries, community mental health centers, counseling agencies and rehabilitation centers, children's homes, and centers for the aging.

Insofar as possible, the CPE student is seen as a co-worker with the other pastoral care staff in these settings. Skill and knowledge are the primary determinants in involvement. For example, at St. Joseph's Hospital in St. Paul, Minn. students often lead the inservice training sessions for our pastoral care staff, because the background of many of these "students" include professional qualifications in such related fields as nursing, medical records, and education.

Other professionals can offer a great deal of valuable input into both staff training and the CPE program. At St. Joseph's Hospital, seminars and workshops are led by professionals in pastoral care and counseling, medicine, psychiatry, nursing, and social service, along with other resource persons from the surrounding community. More informal types of clinical learning also take place.

Actual clinical experience is, of course, the heart of the CPE program. Each student is given clinical responsibility in relation to his ability and interest, and a backup person skilled in pastoral care is assigned to the student as a resource and a model. This kind of program requires careful planning. The individuality of the student must always be respected and opportunities made available that allow for creativity and growth. Thus while one student may need to work with patients on a general medical floor in order to get a "feel" for pain and suffering, another may need to gain creative ministry experience by working with cardiac patients on a specialized unit. Individual research is encouraged in order to fill in gaps in knowledge and understanding.

"Final examinations" are virtually unknown in CPE. Student evaluation is an on-going experience. Each pastoral contact, each report, each group session provides an opportunity to evaluate where the student is and in which direction he needs to go. CPE training is always concluded by an evaluation, but this evaluation is seen more as a statement of where the student *is*, and it is arrived at, in large part, by the input of the student himself. Where each student *is* is always an individual matter.

CPE programs are, of course, concerned with competency, but competency is not assessed only in terms of the number of units completed. Although a given number of CPE units are usually considered necessary, the final evaluation of competence is determined in consultation with both peers and supervisors. Thus a student with only two units of training might wish to be admitted to advanced standing, feeling that sufficient competency has been gained. This judgment may then be confirmed or denied by an advisory committee. But competency, as judged by self, peers, professionals in the field, and supervisors, is the final credential for functioning professionally in pastoral care and counseling. The ability to function in the existential situation is the "final test."

Clinical preparation for pastoral care and counseling, then, as it exists in CPE may be best described as being spiritual-existential-humanistic. It is grounded in the riches of the pastoral care tradition and the resources of the Church; it focuses on the present realities of the moment, promoting awareness and growth; and it underscores, elucidates, and celebrates the humanness of our life experience. It is professional education for ministry.

Confidentiality:
Difficulties in Converting Theory to Practice

LUCIAN A. SAWYER, OSB, BA, B.Th., MA

As any physician or clergyman knows, professional persons have been trained in keeping confidences. The average patient and parishioner takes this for granted, and without another thought, bares his body or soul as the case may be. In this chapter, we will attempt to find the actual roots of confidentiality in theology, on the one hand, and in medicine, on the other. Such an analysis will provide a better perspective on the content of confidential material, the persons involved, and the sharing of information within the spectrum of patient care.

The extension of the doctor's role into a healing team within the hospital makes it imperative that information necessary for the cure of the patient be shared among several individuals. Everyone who is a part of the team has access to information on the patient's chart. This situation makes it virtually impossible to establish principles that will forestall every violation of confidentiality. At best, one can elucidate certain insights that will help team members develop a proper attitude toward patient information.

This chapter deals with confidentiality as it relates to the Pastoral Care Department of a general hospital. However, its principles and conclusions can be applied by all hospital employees where they are relevant to their situations.

A member of a hospital's pastoral care department is the recipient of two long-standing traditions of confidentiality. As a chaplain, he has inherited the tradition of the clergy, with its overtones of "confessional" secrecy; as a hospital team member, he shares the commitment to professional secrecy. This urges upon him a double obligation of discretion.

APPROACHES TO CONFIDENTIALITY

Every textbook on medical ethics or moral theology has a chapter or section on Secrets. While the general statements they make are usually quite clear, the application to life situations demands great discretion.

The question of confidentiality may be studied from two basic perspectives: The first is that of the moral theologian, and the second, that of the medical practitioner. The difference is one of emphasis, since both approaches must overlap.

Roman Catholic theologians, such as Merkelbach, use the expression "secretum commissum" (generally translated as a "professional secret") and treats this subject under the virtue of Justice.[1] His basic assumption is that every man has a right to his own thoughts and to a good reputation, and these two rights are to be respected by everyone else. Information that would hinder these rights should not be divulged. He defines a secret as knowledge of something which is not generally known and must not be made known.

Authors generally distinguish three types of secrets: Natural, promised, and committed. A natural secret is one that by its nature binds us not to reveal something to the disadvantage of another. For instance, if we should discover a "skeleton" in another's family closet, we have a moral obligation not to reveal the information to others, if it is not generally known. This is called "natural" because it grows out of the neighbor's natural right to a good reputation.

A "promised" secret is when we promise someone not to reveal something they have told us. If a friend reveals something very personal about himself and makes us promise not to tell anyone, we are bound not to tell, even if the matter is not hurtful to his reputation.

The third kind of secret is the committed or professional secret. This exists when an implied or explicit contract is made between the owner and the person to whom he reveals personal matter. This is usually the kind of secret involved when the information is necessary for medical treatment or therapy of any kind, and it is the kind that concerns the medical staff and the pastoral care department. In general, theologians teach that secrets of whatever nature are not to be sought, revealed, or taken advantage of without a justifiable reason.

The issue of confidentiality may also be examined from the viewpoint of medical practice. In this context, the preferred textbook word is "confidentiality," rather than "secrecy." The word confidentiality is made up of three Latin roots: "cum" meaning with, "fides" meaning trust, and "litas" meaning state. The emphasis is on the *manner* in which the matter is given (with trust) rather than on the *content* (secret information). This approach finds legal sanction in the American Bill of Rights which guarantees every man's right to privacy. Another legal reinforcement of this approach is found in the *Patient's Bill of Rights*, a statute enacted by the Minnesota Legislature and which reads, "Every patient and resident shall have the right to every consideration of his privacy and individuality as it relates to his social, religious and psychological well being."[2]

A physician is expected to respect a confidence, not exclusively because the information might harm the patient but out of respect for his right to privacy. The Code of the American Medical Association describes what is expected of the physician:

> Patience and delicacy should characterize all the acts of a physician. The confidences concerning individual or domestic life entrusted by a patient to a physician and the defects of disposition or flaws of character observed in patients during medical attendance should be held as a trust and should never be revealed except when imperatively required by the laws of the state.[3]

Trust implies responsibility in the use of information, which can be shared with other members of the healing team, but not revealed publicly without a court order.

The sharing of information is also mentioned in the Nursing Code of 1968, which appears with an official commentary in the *American Journal of Nursing*.[4] "The Nurse safeguards the individual's right to privacy by judiciously protecting information of a confidential nature, sharing only that information relevant to his care."

In summary, theologians approach confidential matter as "hidden knowledge," whereas the medical profession, while not excluding this aspect, emphasizes the "confidential manner" in which the information was given and the responsibility in sharing it.

MATTER INVOLVED

We must distinguish between "confidentiality" which applies to all information imparted by the patient, and "privilege" information, which enjoys the protection of the courts. Those states which have a statute on privilege respect the content of all communication between a doctor and his patient. McFadden delineates what is not privileged communication:

> Only the *content* of the confidential information is covered by privilege. The *fact* that such communication has been made, the *date* thereof, the *number* of consultations or treatments and the *place* and *duration* of treatment do not fall within the privilege.[5]

McFadden places the mantle of ethical responsibility upon all information —

> All confidential information about a patient obtained by a doctor or nurse in the exercise of their medical capacity falls under the medical secret. . . . Not only must medical personnel keep secret confidential information which would slightly or gravely injure the patient if it were revealed, but all confidential information whatsoever must be kept secret. . . . Regardless of what the practice may be, a doctor or nurse may not indiscriminately reveal the secrets of their patients simply because such revelations will not injure the patient. . . . Frequent and unnecessary presumptions upon the consent of the patient are violations of his right to secrecy.[6]

In conclusion, McFadden considers all matter revealed by the patient to be confidential, making allowances for matter not considered "privileged" by the law of the land. Matter on the patient's chart is considered a professional secret and can only be read by those who have a *right* to see it.

Acceptable practice in regard to patient charts for all Catholic institutions was made clear in the American Bishops' Directives: "The charts and records must be duly safeguarded against inspection by those who have no right to see them."[7]

PERSONS

The obligation of confidentiality in matters relating to healing rests primarily upon the doctor, and this obligation can be traced to the Oath of Hippocrates: "Whatever, in connection with my professional practice, or not in connection with it, I may see or hear in the lives of men which ought not to be spoken abroad, I will not divulge, as reckoning that all such should be kept secret."

In the contemporary context, this "secret" becomes a group secret, because such information often must be made available to associate doctors, the operating team, the nurses, technicians, pastoral care, medical records, social service, and members of other departments, the services of which may be needed for efficient health care. Finney and O'Brien trace the line within the group that may share the information: This group, vertical in organization rather than horizontal, should receive only the information needed for the proper performance of their professional or official part in the treatment of the patient."[8]

This "vertical" sharing suggests that the team sharing the information should be structured hierarchically. Confidential information should not be divulged among equals, unless it serves the needs of the particular patient. This leads us to the final point of this study.

USE OF INFORMATION

Theoretical knowledge about confidentiality does not guarantee that the principle will be respected in actual practice. So many human factors enter our everyday social communications that information may drop out which "ought not to be spoken abroad." The habit of discretion must be acquired by personal awareness and by serious reflection following an occasional lapse.

Just as doctors and nurses may share information with others on a professional basis, the same may be said of the members of a hospital pastoral team, who also share responsibility for promoting the patient's welfare. In the course of their duties, members of the pastoral team receive many confidences from the patient. Short of the "confessional seal" which binds the priest, good judgment should be used in sharing information that might help other members in their dealings with the same patient. As always, the norm must be "the benefit of the patient."

When a hospital chaplaincy program includes students in Clinical Pastoral Education, the matter of confidentiality should be discussed early in the program. As part of their training, students must share reports on patients who are actually in the hospital. In these instances, every effort must be made to safeguard the anonymity of the patient, especially in highly personal matters. Farnsworth and Braceland insist that training in confidentiality is necessary. "Indoctrination in the necessity and procedures of confidentiality should be provided at the beginning of seminary training programs in counseling."[9]

Moreover, students should be impressed with the importance of taking care lest they clearly identify patients in their reports.

> Students should not have access to records kept by other students, and highly intimate material should be recorded with as little detail as possible. Indeed, from the earliest stages of their training, counselors should take extreme care to see that only necessary information is included in the record of any client.[10]

Once the anonymity of the patient has been assured, students may present and discuss their reports.

Growth as counselors depends upon reflection and justification of procedures. Common sense should limit the discussions of patients to pertinent times and places. Confidential facts about patients who are presently in the hospital or have recently been discharged should not be discussed with others who are not in the program or in places where the remarks are apt to be overheard.

As was stated at the beginning of this chapter, the principles of confidentiality are quite clear, but no hard and fast rules can apply in every specific case. No matter how technically sophisticated hospital operations become, professional judgment must be used to respect the rights of the individual patient. Bernard Haring summarized the ideal relationship in this simple and moving statement:

> The doctor-patient tie is a covenant of persons. . . . The privacy and intimate reactions of the ailing person transcend by far the impersonal basis of many other relationships. While the seller-buyer contract is founded on com-

mutative justice, the relationship between doctor and patient is distinguished and characterized by such personal attitudes as fidelity, reverence, respect, truthfulness and mutual trust.[11]

FOOTNOTES:

1. Benedictus Henricus Merkelbach, *Summa Theologias Moralis*, Declee de Brouer, Brussels, 1954, Vol. II, p. 820.

2. Statement of Minnesota Statutes, Chapter 688, No. 4, Effective Aug. 1, 1973.

3. *Principles of Medical Ethics*, Guide to Services, American Medical Association, Chicago, 1955, Chap. II, Sec. 2.

4. "Code for Nurses," *American Journal of Nursing*, December, 1968, p. 2582.

5. Charles J. McFadden, *Medical Ethics*, F. A. Davis Co., Philadelphia, 1965, p. 400.

6. *Ibid*, p. 404.

7. *Ethical and Religious Directives for Catholic Health Facilities*, The Catholic Hospital Association, St. Louis, 1971, p. 7.

8. Patrick Finney, CM and Patrick O'Brien, CM, *Moral Problems in Hospital Practice*, Herder, St. Louis, 1956, p. 42.

9. Dana L. Fransworth, MD, and Francis J. Braceland, MD, *Psychiatry, the Clergy, and Pastoral Counseling*, St. John's Press, Collegeville, Minn., 1969, p. 315.

10. *Ibid.*

11. Bernard Haring, *Medical Ethics*, Fides, Notre Dame, Ind., 1973, p. 201.

The Medical Record:

A Valuable Resource for Pastoral Care Persons

SISTER FRANCES JERZAK, SSJ, ART

Have you, as a pastoral care person, ever reviewed a patient's medical record for the purpose of gaining some deeper understanding of the patient and his problems? If the medical record is an unfamiliar reference, you probably feel handicapped in sorting out the information contained in the chart. You may even miss some very helpful facts which would enable you to gain positive insights into the underlying causes of the problem about which the patient consulted you. Your reasons for referring to the chart may be as simple as verifying the patient's age, or as complex as attempting to discover or confirm the behavior pattern and anxieties of a patient faced with a terminal illness.

This chapter develops some basic information about medical records*

---

*My resource for the technical information offered in this chapter is Edna K. Huffman's book, *Medical Record Management*, primarily a basic text for the Registered Record Administrator and the Accredited Record Technician, indicating to them what constitutes an acceptable medical record and detailing what is good medical record management in all its complexities and responsibilities. This is the revised Sixth Edition; the first five were published by Physicians' Record Company under the name of *Manual for Medical Record Librarians*.

We gratefully acknowledge the consultation of Marie C. Dipple, RRA, Director, Medical Record Services, Saint Joseph's Hospital, in the preparation of this material.

and their value to professional pastoral persons who minister to hospitalized patients. It is an attempt to help pastoral care personnel understand the medical record so that they can use it in their role as listener and counselor. The medical record is composed of a multiplicity of forms and reports. Some of these reports, because of their highly technical nature, would be meaningless to those not trained in interpreting them. Needless to say, such reports are of no help to pastoral persons. This chapter will be limited to an examination of those reports which can be helpful to pastoral care personnel.

I do not think it is necessary for pastoral persons to study the medical record of every patient. The medical record ought not to be regarded as a substitute for information volunteered by the patient in personal communication. Rather, it should be used as an additional resource if and when more specific information is needed for effective pastoral contact.

THE MEDICAL RECORD — WHAT IT IS

The medical record is a document that records the hospital experience of the patient from the time of admission until discharge. A complete medical record contains sufficient information to clearly identify the patient, to justify the diagnosis and treatment, and to record the results. A medical record is maintained on every person who has been admitted to the hospital as an inpatient, an outpatient, or as an emergency patient.

PURPOSES OF THE MEDICAL RECORD

The Joint Commission on Accreditation of Hospitals states that the purposes of the medical record are to serve as a basis for planning patient care, to provide a means of communication between the physician and other professionals contributing to the patient's care, and to furnish documentary evidence of the course of the patient's illness and treatment during each hospital admission. It also serves as a basis for analyzing, studying, and evaluating the quality of care rendered to the patient, and provides clinical data for use in research and education. Furthermore, it assists in protecting the legal interests of the patient, hospital, and physician.

CONFIDENTIAL NATURE OF THE MEDICAL RECORD

The information contained in the medical record is acquired in a doctor-patient relationship which is generally considered to be highly confidential or privileged communication. The hospital is responsible for preventing unauthorized persons from gaining access to this medical record from the time the record is initiated, during the hospitalization, and after discharge.

A person involved in pastoral care of the patient can have access to this document in virtue of his role in total patient care. Although he is authorized to review a medical record, he is also under obligation not to divulge any information of a personal nature acquired in the practice of his profession.

Once the patient is discharged, the medical record becomes the custody of the Registered Record Administrator. This highly skilled professional person is responsible for the record in accord with a very definite code of ethics regarding the release of information. Much more can be said about the confidentiality of the medical record; the legal requirements and restrictions regarding it vary from state to state. However interesting though this subject of confidentiality is, it extends beyond the scope of this chapter.

HOW THE MEDICAL RECORD IS BEGUN AND DEVELOPED

The medical record begins in the admitting department at the time of the patient's admission. The essential identification and sociological data is obtained, and this recorded information usually accompanies the patient to the nursing unit. The nurse adds the nurses' bedside record and graphic forms to the record forms received from the admitting office and records how the patient was admitted. The attending physician and his co-workers add their notes. Additional reports are added as they are made.

ARRANGEMENT AND CONTENT OF THE MEDICAL RECORD

The arrangement of the medical record on the nursing unit differs from that used for permanent filing. Here the forms most often referred to during hospitalization are filed in reverse chronological order in the chart holder, from the current date back to the date of admission. During hospitalization, the physician is primarily interested in the condition of the patient and the treatment given between his visits. Consequently, the medical record forms are arranged on the nursing unit according to hospital preference.

At St. Joseph Hospital, St. Paul, Minn., the record, while on the nursing unit, is arranged for easy access to the most recently added information. The chart is separated into five main sections by plainly marked index guides:

1. *Admission Record:* This section contains identification data which is recorded in the admitting office and accompanies the patient to the nursing unit. This section may also contain any special consent forms signed by the patient authorizing specific surgical procedures or treatment.

2. *Nursing Section:* This section records the nurses' observations about the patient, and the nursing care they have given to the

patient. There is also a graphic sheet on which the nurses record the patient's vital signs.

3. *Physicians' Section:* This section contains the history and physical examination, and physicians' progress notes. These comprise a chronological report on the patient, including statements about the patient's clinical course, reaction to treatment, general attitudes affecting treatment, and notations of any changes in treatment. Physicians' orders, surgical reports, and consultation reports by other physicians will be found in this section.

4. *Diagnostic Section:* This section includes the results of all tests which support or justify the final diagnosis, such as laboratory tests, radiology reports, EKG reports, etc.

5. *Therapy Section:* This section records all reports and results of specific therapy given to the patient, such as respiratory therapy, physical therapy, occupational therapy, etc.

One of the most recent additions to the medical forms in use at St. Joseph's Hospital has been a form for "Chaplain's Notes." This was added so that important information, bearing on the care of the patient, might become part of the record. This form is placed immediately prior to the Physician's Progress Notes in the medical record.

After the patient is discharged, his record is transferred to the Medical Record Department for processing and filing. Here, records are arranged into three sections: Identification, medical, and nursing. Within each of these sections, the chart forms are arranged in chronological order for easy review of the medical and clinical data.

**SECTIONS OF MEDICAL RECORD
MOST HELPFUL TO PASTORAL CARE**

Record of Admission (Located in chart, during hospitalization, under *Admission Records)*

This record contains identification data about the patient that will be necessary in recording the administration of Baptism and other Sacraments onto records kept in the pastoral care office. There is a place on this sheet where the priest records the date on which he administered the Sacrament of the Sick. Usually the religious affiliation and parish of the patient is recorded here.

Nurses' Notes (Located in the chart, during hospitalization, under *Nursing Section)*

The nurses' notes record the patient's condition during the physician's absence. Besides being a media of communication between physician and nursing personnel, this acts as proof of work done. During the patient's hospitalization, nurses' notes include daily observations of the patient and a record of medications and treatments given.

At St. Joseph's Hospital, one of the most exciting new methods of recording and arranging patient data has been the emergence of the problem-oriented approach, first introduced by Dr. Lawrence Weed in the late 1950s. Basically, this method contains four elements: 1) Gathering a data base; 2) making up a problem list; 3) drawing up an initial plan of approach; and 4) writing progress notes, each of which is problem-oriented. Some of the advantages of developing such a record are:

1. The problem-oriented method requires a nurse to approach the problems a patient has and to treat them individually in their proper context.
2. This method encourages the nurse to take the initiative in defining and handling problems in the order of their importance.
3. This method allows the physician or those using the record to follow the course of any one problem more easily.

History and Physical Examination (Located in the chart, during hospitalization, under *Physicians' Section*)

The primary purpose of a history and physical examination is to assist the physician in establishing a diagnosis on which to base the care and treatment of the patient. In addition to the history and physical examination, he usually needs the results of laboratory tests and possibly x-rays before he can arrive at a diagnosis. The history should be a record of information provided by the patient. The physical examination is performed after the history has been taken. The format of the history and physical examination will vary according to the style and training of the physician. Basically, and ideally, an acceptable outline for this report would include:

1. Chief Complaint: Brief statement of nature and duration of the symptoms that caused the patient to seek medical attention, as stated in the patient's own owrds.
2. Present Illness: Detailed chronological description of the development of the patient's illness, from the appearance of the first symptom to the present time.
3. Past History: A summary of all illnesses, such as acute infectious diseases, accidents, operations, allergies, drug sensitivites, etc. In women, the number of pregnancies and abortions should be noted.
4. Social History: Statements of marital status, habits, social history, occupation, and environment.
5. Family History: A record of diseases among relatives in which heredity or contact may play a role, such as allergies, infectious disease, mental, metabolic, endocrine, cardiovascular or renal

diseases, or neoplasms. The health of immediate relatives, their ages at death, and causes of death should be recorded.

6. Diagnostic Impression: A tentative or provisional diagnosis made by the physician. This early diagnosis reflects the physician's impression of the patient's condition, but it is made before any of the tests have been completed and a final diagnosis has been reached.
7. Differential Diagnosis: A comparison of symptoms and physical signs of several diseases from which the patient may be suffering. The present illness determines whether or not differential diagnoses are indicated. By the process of elimination of differential diagnoses, the provisional diagnosis may be determined.

Physicians' Progress Notes (Located in the chart, during hospitalization, under *Physicians' Section*)

The physicians' progress notes begin with an admission note, continue with subsequent notes during hospitalization, and conclude with a final note on discharge or death. They give a chronological picture of the patient's clinical course. They are written every day, or even every few hours during the acute phase of the illness, and as often as indicated by the patient's progress thereafter.

Consultation Report (Located in the chart, during hospitalization, under *Physicians' Section*)

A consultant is a second physician, often a specialist, called in by the attending doctor to discuss his patient. Consultations are not necessary in every case. Most commonly, a physician may ask for consultation when the patient is not a good medical or surgical risk, when the diagnosis is obscure, when there is doubt as to the best therapeutic measures to be utilized, in unusually complicated situations where other specific skills may be needed, when the patient exhibits severe psychiatric symptoms, and when it is requested by the patient or his family.

HEALTH RECORD OF THE FUTURE

The newest revolutionary change in medical record science, which is already beginning to take shape in parts of the country and which will eventually involve all health care facilities, is the computerized medical record. The development of this computerized record will require extensive reevaluation of the traditional methods of keeping medical records. Record banks will be built in strategic places around the country. These record banks will contain the complete medical history of all citizens in a particular geographic location from birth to death, and they can be retrieved by health facilities anywhere in the country within minutes. This concept, mind-staggering as it may seem, may pose new problems and new advantages for pastoral care personnel. In the meantime, pastoral persons do have access to information that can be a valuable resource in their specialized ministry.

Patienthood

THE REV. SAMUEL S. KOCHEL, BA, M. Div.

This chapter will investigate the impact that hospitalization has on a person's internal frame of reference. This will be achieved by reviewing the literature and by relating personal experience on the subject of patienthood. This study is not intended to generate findings that can be generalized to all hospitalized persons. Rather, it describes what certain individuals have experienced as their whole existence is changed by confinement to a hospital room and hospital routines. It is intended to heighten the hospital chaplain's awareness of what might be taking place in the patient's internal frame of reference. As will be shown, many individuals have opposite reactions to the hospital environment and routine. Consequently findings cannot be generalized, but they can offer insights into the patient's internal frame of reference, and the chaplain can use these insights when interacting with the patient.

Because this discussion of patienthood presupposes certain principles concerning the nature of man, it is important that these be made explicit for the reader. Each person:

1. Is a unique individual.
2. Experiences his environment in a way that is unique to him.
3. Needs to feel that his existence is important to at least one other person.

4. Needs to be independent and to exercise control over his own life.
5. Needs to feel useful.
6. Has the right to be given intelligible alternatives, on the basis of which he can decide what is most beneficial for him.

From one point of view, patienthood can be described as an intensification and contradiction of the values of our industrial-technical society. As our society shifted emphasis from agriculture to technology, there was a change from a person having relatively unlimited external space and limited internal space to having limited external space and unlimited internal space. A modern day person is physically limited in his ability to view his external world (because of tall, tightly packed buildings), and this sense of limitation is intensified for the hospital patient confined to his room and to what he can actually perceive from his bed. As Kenneth Mitchell relates it: "You lose space. When you're well, your world consists of houses, fields, streets, open spaces, closed spaces — all kinds of space. As a patient, your world is ten feet if you're lucky. It may be even smaller. Your world really shrinks."[1]

The other aspect of space, the internal, is also affected by being a patient. Where internal space can, theoretically, be unlimited for the healthy person, it can be greatly limited for the patient in the hospital. Because of pain, fear of the unknown, and interruption of his daily routine, a person can become almost totally concerned with himself. This can have the effect of making a person lose all interest in what is happening in the world around him.

In addition, the onset of illness and the radical change associated with hospitalization may make a person feel that he has lost his independence and part of his self-worth. As Yehuda Kesten says, "It happened overnight. In one night I changed from a virile, active man to a chronic invalid."[2]

Stewart Alsop relates his feelings about his illness and loss of independence in terms of the contradiction that existed between his family background and life before and after illness and hospitalization. Before, he had been his own master, free to come and go as he pleased. In describing his hospitalization and illness, he states:

"In any case, genes or no genes, the condition to which being seriously ill reduced me was repugnant. I was dependent on the nurses. If I wanted a sleeping pill, or to have my bedclothes changed (I had the sweats every night), I had to ask a nurse. If a nurse woke me up to weigh me, I had to get up and get weighed. It was like being a private all over again.

"I was dependent for my very life on John Glick, and it was he, not I, who decided when I could have my IV removed, whether I could go home, and what I could do when I got there.

"I was dependent above all on Tish, not only for edible and palatable tidbits, books, and the like, but for the squeeze of a warm hand in a season of darkness and fear. Knowing how I resented my state, the emotional sustenance she gave me was always unspoken."[3]

Often, the change in the conditions of modern society and its values caused by hospitalization makes the patient feel like a nonperson. The loss of independence and the diminishing of the cultural values of personhood, of doing, and of achieving have a great impact on a patient. William Sullivan, in a speech to "front line personnel," sponsored by the Twin Cities Council of Hospital Public Relations, said that often he felt like he was treated as a nonperson. He said that the only person who introduced herself was a maid named Ruth. "Never once did I feel anyone took a real interest in me as a person," he said. Rather, he felt as if he was just "another patient to process."[4]

Too often, hospital staff members relate to the patient not in terms of his personhood but in terms of his disease. He is not "Mr. Smith," but rather the "gall bladder in 462." In the case cited above, Mr. Sullivan resented physicians who talked to him as if he were the medical chart rather than a person. He described the experience of being a nonperson as being communicated *at* rather than *to*.[5]

Many studies have been conducted on the attitudes of patients toward their hospital stay. Koos found that 77% of the survey population had negative attitudes towards the care they had received in the hospital. These complaints centered around the depersonalization of the patient. In other words, the dissatisfaction was not with the quality of the care provided in the hospitals, but rather with the manner in which it was provided.[6]

Carl Scherzer characterizes this depersonalization as ego injury in illness. He states that a person in illness undergoes ego injury because of his change in status from being "boss" to being "helpless." The effect of one's illness can cause physical changes, such as confinement to a wheel chair, loss of hair, or loss of strength, all of which conflict with the person's self-concept. Instead of being a person who "does" he may find himself as a person who is done to or done for. Scherzer cites the case of a professional person who was humiliated because he was forced to resort to catheterization for relief.

Conditions which affect a person's appearance also lead to ego injury. Although wearing a brace or being dependent on medication may not, in themselves, cause the patient concern. He may be concerned about the fact that these physical effects of illness might demonstrate his weakness. Scherzer gives many examples of ego injury. It can be expressed by a cantankerous or critical attitude, a simulation of helplessness beyond anything that the condition merits, an oversensitivity to noise or provocation, or a domineering attitude. All of these expressions are attempts to compensate for the feelings of loss of status.[7]

On the other hand, some patients respond in the opposite way. As one woman said, "When I am in here I am the Queen. I can sleep and eat. I don't have to worry about making the bed, cleaning up the house, or fixing the meals. I just push this button and people come to me. Yep, I am a queen. It's like taking a vacation where everything is done for you."

Another element of patienthood can be fear — fear of pain or death, of disfigurement, of the unknown, of the high cost of medical care, of incomplete recuperation from illness, etc. Fear and anxiety are part of a vicious cycle. The patient's unexpressed fear makes it difficult to treat and care for him. He may want assurance, and it may be this very assurance that is so lacking. This lack of assurance makes the patient anxious and he may act erratically which, in turn, frustrates the staff. Thus, patient anxiety and staff anxiety tend to feed each other.[8] Fear may be expressed verbally by direct statements, by asking questions, by demanding attention, or by being critical. It also may be expressed through restlessness, sweating, muscular tension, stomach upsets, diarrhea or constipation, and headaches.[9]

Depending on a patient's condition, he can also suffer the loss of that which gives him pleasure. The effect of pleasure on a person can be a reward or nourishment which stimulates and enhances personal growth. Illness and/or hospitalization interfere with those daily activities that are rewarding and enjoyable. Whether confined to a bed or not, the hospitalized patient is immediately immersed in a routine of activities and services which preclude many of the usual sources of pleasure and gratification.[10] One element of this is not only the isolation from friends and relatives who give pleasure and meaning to life, but also isolation from the sexual routine of sexually active patients. This is most acute in long-term hospitalization.[11]

The last nonphysical aspect of patienthood that we will examine is guilt. Patient guilt may arise from various sources. One writer explains it by saying, "Perhaps the most frequent reason for guilt over incapacitation lies in our moral concepts of role responsibility. A male who is the head of the family, breadwinner, may suffer guilt because he is not working and earning his salary, regardless of whether or not his salary has actually ceased. This feeling is intimately tied to our association of masculinity. . . . For others, the sheer activity itself, the busyness of work, provide a rationale for existence; cessation of work leaves a vacuum to be filled only by inertia and despair. Women also feel a sense of guilt with the clash of the definition of what it means to be a good mother and wife. To be removed from the home for reasons they cannot control becomes a source of guilt."[12]

Guilt can be felt as a punishment for past behavior. It can also arise from a reaction of anger against the "healthy" members of the family and friends who remain undamaged by physical illness. One means of expressing guilt may be through withdrawal and passivity.

There are three elements of the physical environment which occupy a patient's external space: His room, his bed, and the equipment being used in his care. Let us discuss the patient's perception of his room.

Turney Walker describes his room in the following manner: "Your room has four beds, four narrow white cells in the jailhouse of the ward into which you have been locked. . . . You spend a considerable part of your time estimating small but important distances. By the hour, you stare at the open doorway of your room. Somehow, someday, you must walk to that doorway from the faraway pit of helplessness in which you are."[13]

A patient related to me that he lay in his bed and could feel the walls closing in on him. If at other times they didn't seem to be closing in on him, it seemed as if they were going to fall in on him. He went on to say that sometimes he felt like jumping out of his bed and running out of his room because it seemed so small.

Even after a patient realizes that this room is his space, his territory, he has little control over who enters his space. No one knocks or requests to enter the patient's space. In fact, sometimes a patient's room seems like Grand Central Station, with nurses, housekeepers, and doctors coming in and going out whenever they desire.

Kenneth Mitchell calls this a loss of control over who invades your space. He says, "At home, you don't have to let anybody in. Nobody. Unless he has a search warrant. When you're a patient, dozens of people suddenly have a right to come right up to you and touch you and there's nothing you can do about it. Most of them don't even say 'excuse me'."[14]

The second element is the bed. Van Den Berg describes the interrelatedness of the patient and his bed as a conflict. To a healthy person, the bed is a place for sleep and gentleness. To the patient, the bed does not offer a promise of sleep but is a permanent confinement. A healthy person fills his bed with the warmth of his own body. As he lays in his bed he can experience the breeze which brings in the smells of the outdoors, freshness. For the patient, the bed is not a place of experiencing the outside world. The smells of his bed are the specific odor of his sick body. After two or three days the bed has a definite odor. The smell of the sheets, the pillow and pajamas, of everything in close contact with the patient, is a continuous reminder of an existence which knew no changes and which has become stale."[15]

The last area of the physical environment which will be considered is the equipment. Dosia Carlson describes what effect seeing all the equipment had on her: "With all these synthetic pipes, tubes, wires, and catheters winding in and out of the body, many ICU inhabitants looked ready for the launching into orbit. Those with arms or legs rigged up in traction gave even more the appearance of mechanical men. . . . With its chrome and steel trim, our ward in some ways resembled a hardware store."[16]

One piece of equipment which most patients have difficulty dealing with is the bedpan. Not only is it uncomfortable, but it never seems to match the temperature of the body. Patients have reported that they tended to slip off during use. All this spells terror for patients who are required to use them. The "loss of face" syndrome associated with the bedpan comes not only from the physical aspects of the bedpan but also from the feeling that it is taboo to excrete in public. The patient feels that he is violating a social norm and losing his right to privacy and independence.[17]

Faced with the experience of his own hospitalization, the patient often feels broken — broken by loneliness, fear, isolation, separation from friends and family, and conflict with the physical elements of his hospital environment. This brokenness often forces the patient to deal with the basic meaning of life as he interacts in this altered environment with himself, others, and the environment itself. Ashbrook puts it this way: "The very atmosphere of the hospital forces us out of a shell of detachment into the arena of life to wrestle with the basic issues of life and death: Contradictions, meaninglessness, 'internal warfare,' 'guilt and estrangement,' loneliness, anxiety, fear, despair and futility. These feelings comprise the essential components of religious concern."[18]

The chaplain's role is to minister to this brokenness, helping the patient reestablish his wholeness again. Wholeness can be accomplished not only through the physical efforts of all members of the helping professions but by empathetically sharing the patient's internal frame of reference as he deals with brokenness and his search for wholeness. It is most significant that the chaplain can help only if the patient describes his needs and expresses his reactions to his hospitalization.

FOOTNOTES:

1. Kenneth R. Mitchell, *Hospital Chaplain*, Lippincott, Philadelphia, 1972, p. 120.

2. Yehuda Kesten, *Diary of a Heart Patient*, D. Van Norstrand, New York City, 1968, p. 2-3.

3. Stewart Alsop, *Stay of Execution*, Lippincott, Philadelphia, 1973, p. 253.

4. Cynthia Boyd, "Being Treated as a Nonperson Called Worst Hospital Experience," *St. Paul Pioneer Press*, May 24, 1974, p. 14.

5. *Ibid.*

6. Lewis Bernstein and Richard Dana, *Interviewing and the Health Professions*, Appleton Century Crofts, New York City, 1970, p. 7.

7. Carl J. Scherzer, "Ego Injury in Illness," *Pastoral Psychology*, April, 1975, p. 31-34.

8. Clyde Schallenberger, "I'm Frightened," *Alumnae Magazine*, Johns Hopkins School of Nursing, Sept. 1970, p. 56.

9. Bernstein and Dana, *op. cit.*, p. 120.

10. *Ibid.*, p. 122-123.

11. Wayne Oates, "The Inner World of the Patient," *Pastoral Psychology*, April 1975, p. 16-17.

12. Bernstein and Dana, *op. cit.*, p. 129-130.

13. Twinley Walker, *Rise Up and Walk*, E. P. Dutton, New York City, 1950, p. 11, 24.

14. Mitchell, *op. cit.*, p. 120.

15. J. H. Van Den Berg, *The Psychology of the Sickbed*, Duquesne, Pittsburgh, 1967, p. 61-65.

16. Dosia Carlson, *The Unbroken Vigil*, John Knox, Richmond, 1968, p. 78.

17. Barbara Nelson, "Why Patients Hate Bedpans," *Modern Healthcare*, June, 1974, p. 48-50.

18. Virginia Nehring and Barbara Geach, "Patient's Evaluation of Their Care, Why They Don't Complain," *Nursing Outlook*, May, 1973, p. 3.

Pain

SISTER RITA RIORDAN, CSJ, BA
SISTER ANN MICHELE JADLOWSKI, CSJ, BA, MA

According to Aristotle, pain is the antithesis of pleasure, the epitome of unpleasantness. A common definition of pain used today is unpleasant or distressing physical sensation due to bodily injury or disorder, or acute mental or emotional distress or suffering. The very word pain is derived from the Latin root *poena*, meaning penalty or punishment.

Clinically, pain consists of two elements: Sensation and reaction to sensation. The second element is more complex, because it involves both physical and emotional reaction and thus engages the highest mental functions of the patient.

Pain has multiple areas of involvement: Physical, neurological, behavioral, psychiatric, etc. Superficial kinds of pain can be fairly easily defined. For example, the patient can locate the organ and describe the pain as sharp, burning, shooting, etc. However, so-called visceral pain is more difficult to describe. It may be nagging, spreading, aching; at the same time, it may be difficult to locate specifically. Every organ of the body can make itself felt through the pain experience.

Intensity of pain depends largely on temporary environmental influences or on the person's state of consciousness. For example if a person is in a state of shock, perhaps as a result of an accident, often he will not feel pain until sometime later, perhaps not until hospitalization has occurred. Any high emotional involvement may tend to repress or reduce pain, by shifting the patient's concentration to something other than the pain and thereby reducing the experienced intensity of the pain. Sometimes the patient himself will turn to some physical activity such as shouting, crying, fist clenching, or teeth grinding for distraction from the intense pain.

Although few experiences in life are as universal as pain, it seems one of the most difficult to describe. Pain can interfere with every aspect of living; with work, play, eating, sleeping, praying, visiting, listening. Some people have a high threshold for pain, some do not. Generally speaking, a person with an apathetic, stoic temperament has a higher threshold than the person who is high-strung or nervous, or who is experiencing a period of strong emotional stress. Also, it is generally true that as pain becomes more severe in one area it usually becomes less in another.

Since there is no really accurate way to judge the degree of pain which a person may be experiencing, it is best to take the person's word for it. Perhaps nothing can anger a person in pain more than to be told that he "really doesn't feel that pain." While in general no one ever becomes really used to pain, it is also true that tolerance to pain often increases in some individuals, while it decreases in others.

Pain differs from patient to patient and in any given patient from time to time. Night is usually the time that pain seems to be worse, perhaps due to the fact that this is often the loneliest time and the patient tends to experience more fear and anxiety. Actually, he may not be experiencing greater pain, but rather a stronger reaction to it.

There are many variables related to the perception of and reaction to pain, including the person's emotional state, the knowledge he has of his condition, and any past experiences related to his particular pain. For example, does his headache remind him of the headaches his grandfather had prior to his fatal stroke? Another variable that affects the patient's pain level is the degree of confidence he has in his medical team. Since fear and anxiety affect pain, the patient's confidence in his doctor or medical team may help to diminish fear and anxiety.

Pain has been part of man's experience for all time. In Genesis 3:16 we read: "I will multiply your pain in childbearing. You shall give birth to your children in pain." Jeremiah, referring to communal rather than individual pain, says: "Why bother to complain about your wound? Your pain is incurable." In the lifetime of Christ, many people suffered pain both from disease and from emotional stress. Jesus is always the healer except when it comes to his own pain, which he bears. "The Son of Man is destined to suffer grievously. . . ." Luke 9:22. "They twisted thorns into a crown and put it on Him . . . struck his head with a reed. . . . It was the third hour when they crucified him." Mark 15:16ff.

For thousands of years, man thought of pain as punishment for moral depravity and wickedness. Until recently, Christianity taught the opposite, i.e., that bearing pain strengthens the will, regulates the passions, and leads to God. Although there may be much wisdom in this interpretation, it is extremely hard to justify it in the light of the teachings of Jesus. Certainly there is pain connected with moral depravity and certainly wisdom may be increased through suffering, but there is also much pain and suffering that bear no relation to depravity and wickedness and which do not lead to either wisdom or God.

Our generation and the preceding two have heard much about the conflict between science and religion. Religion has realized that it cannot provide all the answers to the question, "Why does pain exist?" Science is learning that it does not have all the answers either. Although the radical advances in the control of pain are much to be applauded, mere technical competence in this area is not enough. Many people feel that religion and medicine may find that this phenomenon of pain provides a real point of interaction and service that may have many benefits for those they seek to serve. The patient always receives a greater benefit when he is treated according to a "wholistic" approach.

Part of the problem in the treatment of pain is that it is still too little understood. That pain is indeed mystery becomes more obvious when we note that however and to whomever it comes, it is an event. Often it hits suddenly, from natural causes and disasters, or from historical causes. However it comes, it is real, it is tragic, and it can render us silent and numb. It often imparts to us a sense of awesome mystery that is hard to articulate.

How does man respond to pain? Paul Lindell[1] tells us that some attempt to avoid it through drugs, anesthesia, acupuncture, apathy, or noninvolvement. Others try the route of radical endurance, deliberately trying to reason out a logical and controlled response. Still others rebel against it by turning to various modes of destructive bitterness.

For the Christian, none of these attempts at dealing with the mystery will bring peace and none is redemptive. To attempt to avoid or to remain stoic or to rebel simply confronts one type of pain with another. In none of these reactions will man find a Savior who has spoken a message of a new creation, of healing and restoration through His own death and resurrection. Following the example of Jesus, the redemptive experience can only be achieved when there is involvement, confrontation, a willingness to live with what is unknown, and when there is an allowance for strength and power that comes from beyond the person. Many patients have reported a feeling of having almost literally a "new life" following intense suffering and pain.

Brena[2] has raised some interesting questions about the long-range involvement of organized religious institutions in programs of psychophysical rehabilitation. (It isn't clear if he has any knowledge of modern hospital pastoral care.) He asks whether it is realistic to anticipate an efficient collaboration between the religious and health professions at the patient's bedside? He testifies to the value of priest-physician teamwork with drug dependency and wonders whether this approach would also help the patient suffering physical pain. Asking if pain is necessary in the life of humans, his answer seems to be yes and no: Yes, because pain is a useful warning signal and an imperative behavior provider in the face of injury or disease, which we could hardly survive without. It is also necessary, because we can be helped to use pain as blessing. No, because it is an artifact of our imperfect nature.

Lindell[3] addresses himself to the blessing of pain. How can blessing flow from pain? Pain may be a cleansing experience, bringing the person closer to Christ. It can make us more intensely aware of our call to reflect the life of the Son of God in our own bodies, to walk as Jesus did. Often our days become distorted and events fall out of focus; how quickly, though, realities fit together for us when pain redirects our vision to really important things. The Apostle Paul, writing often of his own sufferings, reminds us that in sufferings we learn to comfort others who are in pain around us. Pain can affect our worship, as it did the worship of Job. Not only can it affect the sufferer's worship, but pain can also move those who observe the loved one to call out: "Out of the depths I cry to Thee, O Lord." Psalm 130:1

What are some of the ways that those in pastoral care work can help the patient? In the first place, they can show their interest and concern by being present, by being aware of where the patient is, by responding to his loneliness, and actually contributing to the relief of pain. The fight against pain is carried on in different levels: Physical and pharmacological treatment, surgical treatment, and psychological treatment. Psychological healing takes place primarily in the interaction between the patient and the treatment team. When that team includes someone trained in professional pastoral care, the psychological treatment can be greatly facilitated. No one is in a better position to give comfort and consolation than pastoral care professionals.

In terms of specific approaches to use in the presence of pain, pastoral personnel believe that it is helpful to assist the sufferer to accept his pain as true and real. I can make the words of the Apostle Paul my own, "For the sake of Christ then, I am content with weaknesses, insults, hardships, persecutions, and calamities." By itself, pain is real, actual, harsh, cruel, and destructive. But it can be turned into something quite different through acceptance — not in a passive way, but in an active way that wrestles the blessing from it. Pastoral ministers must be encouraged to follow the example of Jesus in his public ministry, and tackle the problem of pain. In so doing, they must use whatever tools are at hand — the medications, the surgical procedures, rest, food, etc. These are the instruments of the new creation.

There is another dimension to the problem of pain which I would also like to point to here. As the dimension of pain exists for the stricken person, so there is pain in the heart of the person who attempts to move toward a healing of that pain. Thus, pain becomes a reality for the minister, and for him to be truly "healer" he must face his own pain and make some decisions about it. If the minister is to understand pain, in relation to those to whom he ministers, he must first come to understand the pain in his own life and be at peace with himself. In other words, he can face in others only what he has faced in himself.

To be authentically involved in another's pain, we must first answer some questions for ourselves. How we answer these questions will determine, in large part, whether we enter a pain-filled situation with great difficulty or too easily, or whether we enter as true pastoral ministers capable of empathy with the person in pain. Some of the questions that we must ask ourselves have been suggested by James Ashbrook[4]: 1. Do I want to help? 2. Am I tough enough to get involved in another's pain? 3. Am I humble enough? These questions are broad in scope. For example, given differing personalities, value systems, needs, do I honestly want to get involved in a particular situation? And, just how tough am I? Can I allow my path, my uniqueness, my life style to clash with that of the sufferer and still survive as a person myself? It takes toughness to keep returning to a bedside and risking rejection, when your heart says, "go back, just try to be a presence," and your legs say, "let's get out of here." Do I understand humility rightly? Is there an appropriateness about me, my own life, my own needs? Can I be fulfilled with the realization that I have only a part of an answer to pain?

We cannot answer these kinds of soul-searching questions without experiencing pain. Nor can we answer them by ourselves. In our need, we find ourselves turning to Him, who alone can give meaning to our pain and help us share this meaning with those to whom we minister.

The pain experience will continue to be part of the human condition, at least into the foreseeable future. Although science continually attempts to relieve the suffering caused by pain, it is important to remember that relief is facilitated and the acceptance of pain made more attainable through the empathetic sharing of others.

We find the beginning of "pain" in Genesis and we find the end in Revelations:

> "Behold, the dwelling of God with men. He will dwell with them and they shall be his people; and God himself will be with them; He will wipe away every tear from their eyes and death shall be no more; neither shall there be any mourning, nor crying, nor pain any more, for the former things have passed away." Rev. 21:3-4

FOOTNOTES:

1. Paul Lindell, *The Mystery of Pain*, Augsburg Publishing House, Minneapolis, 1974.

2. Steven F. Brena, *Pain and Religion: A Psychophysiological Study*, Charles C. Thomas, Springfield, Ill., 1972.

3. Lindell, *op. cit.*

4. James Ashbrook, *Responding to Human Pain*, Judson Press, Valley Forge, Pa., 1975.

Spiritual Therapy for the
Person in Isolation

SISTER AGNES REINERT, OSB, RN

My personal clinical experience has convinced me that the person in isolation presents the pastoral care person with a unique opportunity for a specific kind of ministry. In my own experience, the knowledge that I would be working with a person who was in isolation led to a certain feeling of constraint. Even though nonisolation contacts have proven more challenging than a second or third contact, I was aware of feeling less free to risk involvement in cases where the initial contact was to take place in the isolation set-up. These specific contacts created a seemingly greater emotional distance in me. Consequently, in this chapter, my objective is, first, to attempt to understand whether the person in isolation has unique feelings about being in this protective set-up and, second, to establish what implications the person's needs have as regards the pastoral minister.

The principle underlying the rationale for protective care is expressed in the definition of communicable disease: "A communicable disease is one which can be transmitted, directly or indirectly, from one person to another. Several of the communicable diseases are caused by some form of virus."[1] Therefore, it seems imperative that all professional persons having relationships with the patient in isolation be informed regarding the nature of the disease for which the patient is in isolation so as to take appropriate preventive measures. These basic measures. These basic measures include the use of an isolation gown, a mask which covers the nose and mouth, and hand-washing immediately after taking off the gown and leaving the room. These precautionary measures are prescribed by the mode of transmission of many communicable diseases. Since many pathogenic organisms are air-borne or thrive in warm, moist skin areas, a visitor — merely by shaking hands with the patient — could very easily and unknowingly transmit a disease to self and to others if he failed to observe precautionary preventive measures.

Another helpful principle that pertains to isolation states: "To prevent or control transfer of infection and disease, all individuals known to be affected by, or to be harboring or producing the pathogenic organisms, must be separated from others. This separation of the patient or affected person from others is termed isolation."[2] The length of time the affected person must be isolated depends on the incubation period of the disease, the length of time the disease is infectious or transmissible, whether the person becomes a carrier, and the time in isolation that may have been established through medical research of the disease in the past.[3]

The patient in isolation for communicable disease faces special emotional problems. Studies on sensory deprivation show that patients deprived of the stimulation of contact with others may quickly become prey to frightening fantasies. Every effort should be made to maintain contact with the isolated person and especially to express continued acceptance of him as a person, and not to react negatively toward him because of his condition.[4]

The psychological needs of the person in isolation are, basically, the same needs of every person but often more intensified. This is especially true of the need to love and to be loved and the need to feel that one is worthwhile to one's self and to others.[5]

At this point I would like to illustrate the experience of the person in isolation by reference to five "living human documents" with whom I had contact.

Contact A: Mrs. P is a 71-year-old woman who was hospitalized for six weeks. During her stay, she was isolated until three days before her discharge from the hospital, because of an open lesion on the side of her ankle which was draining. A circulatory problem in her legs confined her to bed for the first four weeks of her stay. During the fifth week, she was permitted to get up only to use the bathroom located in her own room. Some of the comments this woman made during her hospitalization were most meaningful in helping me understand what the person is actually feeling and thinking while in isolation:

"I feel confined being in this room. I can't go out."

"The food isn't interesting on paper plates. Once in a while wouldn't be bad, but every meal, every day; and the hot food isn't hot and the cold food isn't cold. It gets so monotonous."

"I feel some of my relatives are afraid to come. Last week my 18-year-old grandson wanted to kiss me goodbye; I had to tell him he couldn't — that hurt me and it was hard for him too; we're such an affectionate family. I see physical closeness to be a problem for me being in isolation, but I can still feel emotionally close to people."

"My friends would come more freely if I weren't in isolation."

"The nurses have been very good. They are really comfortable in coming in and taking care of me."

"My hardest thing is the boredom and monotony of being in bed. I'm not able to pray. I can't read much. I think about dying (breaks into tears and sobbing). I'm frightened, especially at night. I've thought about death at home but now I have so much time to think about myself. . . I don't like this. I'd rather cover it up and put it out of my mind."

"I'm always glad to see someone. Visiting has been the biggest help to me while in here. The phone calls have been helpful to me, too."

Contact B: Mr. B is a 32-year-old man who has an infection in his hand which resulted from an earlier cut sustained at his place of work. He has been in isolation since admission, which is about one week. In comparing his present situation with a former hospitalization during which he was not in isolation, he says:

"I feel there is less contact with persons; people go back and forth outside my door but don't seem to want to come in."

"The thing that is hard for me is not being able to go out in the hall and visit other patients."

"My buddy was really uncomfortable with that gown-bit. I had to tease him into actually putting it on."

"I've watched enough TV for the rest of my life. I'm TV'd to death here, but I watch it to get rid of the monotony of these four walls. The social contacts by phone are my life-savers. I really like the interaction I have with the nurses and my visitors; it helps me to feel more in touch with what is going on outdoors."

Contact C: This middle-aged man, who came daily to see his mother who was in isolation because of an infected toe, had this to say from the visitor's point of view:

"I sure don't feel free to come in and go out of this room as I'd like to. These gowns are so awkward to wear. I can't get comfortable with wearing them."

Contact D: Mr. D is 74 years old and is hospitalized in isolation for gangrene of his foot with an accompanying ulceration of the toe that is a staphlococcal infection. He is scheduled to have his leg amputated in a couple of days. When asked what his feelings were in regards to being in isolation, he responded:

"It's all right with me. I don't mind. I live alone and manage for myself. I don't think I can manage after this surgery though."

"I was in an isolation room the last time, too. That was a year ago when I had to have the other leg amputated."

Contact E: Mrs. E, an 84-year-old woman, has a skin and tissue breakdown with underlying infection. She has been in isolation now for five weeks and frequently expresses a desire to sleep during daytime hours. After being with her for 20 minutes, during which time we shared silences and small talk and more serious talk in which she raspily said that she felt her body was "about worn out," she continued to share her personal feelings and fears while clinging to my hand. Three times in the course of this sharing, she made the statement: "It's good to know someone cares." She also commented, "I'm afraid and I feel alone so much of the time."

These five contacts, each of which is unique, offer opportunities for pastoral care. *Contact A* was able to express her fears regarding death. Once she had expressed this fear and realized that she was being accepted and understood, she seemed less tense and discouraged during the remainder of her stay in the hospital. She welcomed visitors and recognized her need to share in relationship with other persons.

Contact B was finding his situation somewhat confining, both physically and socially. He admitted being uncomfortable when alone and that he filled up the silence with TV and phone calls. He appreciated social contacts and also wanted to experience human relatedness and to maintain an interest in the outside world.

Contact C, the visitor in an isolation room, had a need to be understood and accepted for how he felt about his involvement and responsibility toward the patient in isolation. *Contact D* seemed to expect to be in isolation and to accept it. His situation was unique in that his self-image was forcibly being threatened by a second amputation of a limb. He needed to know that he was accepted and loved as a person, whole, worthwhile, and possessing dignity.

Contact E's statement of feeling so alone and so afraid was an open invitation for a caring person to be present to her. Her statement, "It's good to know someone cares," made me feel that I didn't need to search for further resources at this time, since my presence was enough.

In general, as a result of pastoral visits, each of these five individuals was able to take a closer look at his situation in order to evaluate it, to become more aware of his own feelings about being in isolation, and to be better able to express these feelings, i.e., the fear of death, the fear of becoming increasingly dependent, the fear of being alone, and the need to see and talk to people.

One feeling common to all these persons was the feeling of aloneness and the experience of loneliness. Ira Tanner has developed a concept to explain a person's feelings in relation to being alone.[6] He says that it is not surprising for people to dread being alone, because then all one has is one's self. Being alone allows unpleasant feelings of fear, inadequacy, anger, guilt, discontent, or helplessness to surface. If these feelings are intense enough, the person views times of aloneness as unwelcome and even frightening intervals.

Almost everything in life is geared toward togetherness, and people seldom allow themselves time to experience aloneness. Being alone with one's self is to be alone with one's own thoughts and feelings. If the person likes and accepts his thoughts and feelings, aloneness can be a good experience, but if one does not like them, his aloneness can be frightening.

If the person is alone, not by choice but because of circumstances, such as a specific illness or disease over which he has little or no control, he has the option of accepting the aloneness experience. Such acceptance can serve ultimately to bring out the person's best possibilities. It offers the individual time in which to evaluate his personal goals, the quality of his work, his values and faith, and it can lead him to a new appreciation of his relatedness to spouse, friend, or God.

We feel important to the person who "works" to understand us. Understanding is the most valuable gift one person can give another, because the cost is the giving of one's self. In relation to others, the opposite of loneliness is understanding. Understanding thaws loneliness.

To share feelings is to share the most personal component of one's self. Feelings lie at the core of the person and hence are shared in a very selective manner so that the person reduces the "risk" to self. In the process of working to understand another person, the pastoral person becomes more in touch with his personal feelings. Both persons involved in the relationship experience new energy beginning to flow within themselves, and they begin to realize that their interchange has brought each of them more to life and more in touch with their own inner resources.

Some persons seem more lonely than others. This feeling of loneliness hinges on the intensity of the person's fear of love.[7] "Nothing soothes and complements an individual's need for love more than a touch." In fact, the lessening of physical contact with others contributes to many persons' loneliness pain.[8]

In the description of the five persons quoted above, each expressed a need for relatedness in their aloneness. They are asking for support for their sense of dignity and integrity in an effort to maintain feelings of humanness and wholeness. In the more intense hours of loneliness, and in the experience of isolation, the person comes to realize the treasure of the human voice, the beauty of the smile, and the wonder and glowing fulfillment of human relatedness.[9]

Being a pastoral care person has enabled me to take a closer look at what my role and identity mean to the person in isolation. I am aware of being recognized as representing the Church, and I feel this asset allows me to affirm the value of life and of humanness on a deeper level than I could through any other identification. I can reassure the person that he or she is valuable through the relatedness established in ongoing contacts. Also, my identification with religion can be a facilitating agent, because religion can call forth the person's own resources in confronting the problems inherent in their unique situation.

More specifically, the role of the pastoral care person would be to express care and concern for the person in isolation. In the course of these contacts, the patient realizes the value of the caring person's presence and feels free to express frightening fears. The understanding that is established enables the patient to affirm his or her own worth, thus bringing him closer to the fulness of health. Knowing the principles related to isolation, the pastoral worker should feel free to use touch as a means of expressing concern to the person in isolation.

FOOTNOTES:

1. Alice L. Price, *The Art, Science, and Spirit of Nursing*, W. B. Saunders Co., Philadelphia, 1965, p. 453.

2. *Ibid.*, p. 456.

3. *Ibid.*

4. Arthur Noyes, William Camp, and Mildred Van Sickel, *Psychiatric Nursing*, MacMillan Company, New York City, 1964, pp. 285, 286.

5. William Glasser, *Reality Therapy*, Harper & Row Publishers, New York City, 1965, p. 9.

6. Ira Tanner, *Loneliness: The Fear of Love*, Harper and Row Publishers, New York City, 1965.

7. *Ibid.*, p. 3.

8. *Ibid.*, p. 18.

9. Clark E. Moustakas, *Loneliness*, Prentice-Hall., Inc., Jersey, 1961, p. 60.

Psychological Effects of Congenital Anomalies Upon Parents and Siblings

FATHER JAMES PICCHIARINI, BA

In this chapter, I would like to investigate what happens psychologically/emotionally to parents and siblings when a special child, a child with a congenital birth defect, is born into their family. Secondly, I would like to explore the question of what the helping professions can do to help families in this difficult time.

When parents hear the words, "Your baby is defective," life does indeed stand still for them. At that moment, they cannot begin to understand the ramifications of the news they hear. Their life will be unalterably changed. The psychological, physical, emotional, financial, spiritual, and social health of the family is at stake.

The emotional reactions of parents depend upon many variable factors,[1] the combinations of which are unique with each family. Some of these factors are:

1. The parents' own temperaments, personality adjustments, degree of flexibility, patterns of dealing with crises, and attitudes and prejudices. Some parents have sufficient understanding, emotional stability and whatever else it takes to cope fairly adequately with the problem. Others seem to lack these qualities and meet the situation inadequately. One set of parents may care

profoundly and another may appear quite indifferent. Some self-centered parents simply do not care enough, and are unwilling to adjust their lives and rearrange their priorities. In short, the emotional health factor of the parents is an important variable. Are they healthy and stable emotionally? What are their own attitudes toward the mental or physical handicap of their child?

2. The type and extent of the defect. Feelings about bodily deformity or facial disfigurement are generally more intense than are those toward a physical handicap which is not immediately apparent, for example, speech or hearing disorders, convulsive seizures, heart defects, or diabetes.

3. Prognosis. The prognosis will determine how long deprivations and sacrifices have to be endured by the family. Usually, it conforms to one of the following:

   a. Conditions that are irreversible and mean early death.

   b. Conditions which require long-term, costly treatment.

   c. Conditions involving lifelong disability, with all the accompanying fears about education, vocational choice, marriage, and the future.

4. Religious differences. This variable includes the presence or absence of spiritual strengths and resources in the parents.

5. Family's position in the community and their ambitions to reach certain goals.

6. Special meanings children have for their parents. Pride in one's children and anticipation of high achievement by a child are two special meanings children have for their parents.

7. Society's demand for perfection, success, and achievement. Our society places a premium on appearance, higher education, artistic skills, and special abilities. Parents are caught up with this factor in varying degrees. Are they success and achievement-oriented people to the degree of being insensitive to a physical or mental handicap?

With such wide variations among families, as well as among birth defects and the situations in which they occur, it may appear impossible that anything common in the emotional reactions of parents to their deformed children would surface. However the reverse is true.

THE THREE STAGES

Evelin Jacobs, a social worker and program consultant for the National Society for Crippled Children and Adults, has outlined three stages[2, 3] through which parents pass before reaching some kind of acceptance of their disabled child. These three stages include:

Stage 1 — Emotional Disorganization/Shock and Mourning Period.

Stage 2 — Emotional Reintegration/Search or Determination Period.

Stage 3 — Mature Adaptation/Recovery Period.

Let us examine each of these in detail.

Stage 1

As mentioned above, the first stage is a stage of emotional disorganization or a period of shock and mourning. When parents first hear the news that their child is not right, the main reactions are shock, disbelief, and disappointment, accompanied by varying degrees of embarrassment, resentment, hostility, anger, shame, guilt, confusion, and anxiety.

Although during pregnancy, most parents consider the possibility something might go wrong or that their child might be abnormal, the overriding feeling during this time is one of hopeful expectation. Preparations are made for the baby's arrival. The crib is set up, baby clothes are considered, and the nursery is decorated. If the pregnancy is wanted and planned, the nine months are full of pleasure and joy.

With the birth of the abnormal child, the parents are shocked by the shattering of their hopes and dreams. A defective birth differs basically from the other two great misfortunes of life, namely ill health and death. We are accustomed to living with the realities of sickness and death and not only the parents, but the helping professions as well, are much better equipped to deal with these realities than with what might be called a living death, the birth of an abnormal infant. The birth of a defective child bears similarity to death insofar as both involve feelings of loss: Intense longings for the desired child; resentment of the cruel blow that life's experience has dealt. The great and far-reaching difference between the two lies, so to speak, in the continuing presence of this death, day after day. Burial of a dead child gives some finality to this trauma, but the defective child is present, day by day, to renew the trauma.

The obvious feelings expressed at this time — feelings of shock, disbelief, and disappointment — can be readily understood. However, other feelings may surface which require more subtle understanding. The most commonly asked question is, "Why?" or "What caused this?" Linked to this question may be strong anxiety feelings about the biological inadequacy of the parents. The parents might really be asking, "What's the matter with us as propagators?"

The mother especially may feel a failure to produce what she has long prepared herself to create. The birth may be a threat to her sense of adequacy and worth and a threat to her femininity. Cultural and societal pressures come to bear. Our society sets rigid standards of appearance and intellectual functioning, and the parents' anxiety about the child's birth is related to their ego status.

Then the old bugaboo of guilt, real or imagined, can rear its ugly head. Parental feelings of guilt-punishment are not uncommon. Imagine the parent's possible guilt if, in the first place, they rejected the pregnancy. They could very well feel that they are being punished for not wanting the baby. The mother who has attempted an unsuccessful home remedy abortion and then gives birth to an abnormal child shows much guilt in her reaction to the child. The guilt grows out of her fear that, in attempting to destroy the child, she has harmed him. If she sees the baby as an extension of herself, her guilt will make her feel that she has given birth to a "bad" part of herself for everyone to see.

As parents wrestle with the question "Why," they scrutinize their past lives for any sins they may have committed or mistakes they have made. Besides initial rejection of the pregnancy, other incidents to which guilty feelings can be attached are premarital sex, masturbation, venereal disease, and extra-marital relationships.

Anger is another common emotional reaction, anger against God or fate. This anger can be directed against God's official representative, the hospital chaplain, or against doctors or nurses. Often the question that is asked is "Why did God do this to me?"

An additional emotional response on the part of the parents may be for one to blame the other because of previous disease or some hereditary factor on one side of the family, possibly a similar abnormality in an aunt or uncle or some other relative. The parents will probably also inquire about the likelihood of a similar abnormality occurring in their next child.

Denial is a defense mechanism used sometimes by parents during this first stage. Basically, denial is the inability to acknowledge the real situation because it is extremely painful. As do all defense mechanisms, denial serves a useful function initially until the parents can muster their resources sufficiently to deal with reality. Grief work over the loss of the expected normal child must be done and all the initial feelings already mentioned must be expressed. However, prolonged denial in the face of evidence to the contrary is certainly an unhealthy sign.

Another practical question in this first stage is "Should the parents see the child?" This is a very sensitive issue. Susanne Kohut, social worker, points out that parents may question their tolerance for seeing the child. Sometimes well-intentioned doctors, wishing to spare the parents any further pain, may advise the parents not to see the child. This advice may compound the parents' problems. Coming from professionals who supposedly have seen everything in the way of birth defects, this advice confirms the fears of the parents that they have produced a terrifying monster. Secondly, not seeing the child may reinforce the guilt the parents already feel, since this decision conflicts with society's expectations of parental behavior.[4] Refusal to see a child is an act of extreme rejection, the guilt and consequences of which may haunt parents for the rest of their lives.

Stage 2

Hopefully, with time and much support from caring professionals, the parents will move to the second stage of their adaptation. This stage is called the stage of reintegration or the search or determination stage. The primary question at this stage is not "Why?" but "What can be done?" At this time, the parents learn about their child's condition and about what realistic expectations they can have for their child. This is the time for evaluating the child's prognosis.

In regard to prognosis, Park White says:

"In view of the marvelous advances in plastic surgery, we may divide congenital malformations into those about which something definite can be done and with every hope of success; those about which something can and should be done, the success of which is doubtful; and those about which, in all honesty, nothing can or should be done save only adjustment, 'learning to live with it.' "[5]

He goes on to say that the first or readily reparable group includes such conditions as harelip, cleft palate, certain types of birthmarks, clubfeet, and most congenital hernias. Among the more serious and possibly reparable defects are exstrophy of the bladder, congenital cataract, certain operable heart abnormalities, and various types of intestinal obstructions. Finally, there are the heart-rendering cases where the child is irremediably malformed or retarded. This group includes mongolism, cerebral palsy, blindness, and inoperable heart conditions.

After the type of anomaly is determined, the question most parents ask is, "What can be done and how soon?" It is extremely difficult, though often necessary, to accept the fact that nothing at all should be done immediately. It is hard for parents to accept a delay in treatment, but waiting to see how nature will care for the situation may well be the best course. Often, the parents are tempted to go doctor shopping or clinic shopping, to their emotional and financial detriment. It is not unknown for parents to resort to quackism if a quack will tell them what they want to hear.

Another critical area that must be dealt with in this searching stage is the immediate planning for the baby. What happens when the doctor says, "Your baby is ready for discharge"? The parents' response may be one of alarm and confusion. They may wonder why the hospital cannot keep the baby indefinitely. To decide whether to institutionalize the baby or take the baby home is always a painful and difficult decision for parents to make. They must consider whether they are able to give the baby the care it needs at home and whether the family, especially if there are other children, can remain emotionally healthy when their entire pattern of living may have to change.

On the other hand, there is the social and cultural pressure upon parents to assume the obligation of caring for their children. Susanne Kohut[6] says:

"The final decision as to where the child goes will depend on a number of factors. How concerned are the parents about the child and how well do they perceive his needs? Is there sufficient strength in the family to cope with the problem in a mutually supportive way?"

She continues:

"Sometimes realistic difficulties — such as crowded housing conditions, absence of the father, or illness or frailty of the mother — may stand in the way of taking the child home. Studies have shown that the degree of social disorganization in the home has significant correlation with the quality of care the child will receive. In the presence of serious social pathology, placement must be considered to protect the well-being of the child. However, the presence of poverty alone need not prevent good paternal care."

If the decision is made to keep the child at home, a whole new constellation of problems await the parents and other family members. There are the practical problems of lifting, toileting, and feeding a handicapped child. Mary Marguerite Matheny[7] describes the task of a mother of a handicapped child:

The mother, who is conscientiously trying to follow all the instructions of well-meaning therapists and teachers, suddenly finds herself trying to be a physical therapist, an occupational therapist, a speech therapist, an educator, a nurse, a wife to her husband, a mother to her other children, a cook for the family, a maid, a housekeeper, a laundress, Still she is expected to do her share of church work, to be a den mother and to assume her share of responsibility to the community.

Under this pressure, a mother can easily explode in anger, bearing resentment toward her child. Anger toward those one loves produces guilt, and this guilt can be compounded when one is angry and resentful toward a child whose handicap is beyond his control.

Marital relationships also become strained. The mother will carry the major burden of caring for her handicapped child. The father can understandably feel guilty about this or possibly because of his secret feeling of relief that it is his wife and not he who has to carry the burden. The strength of the marital relationship is of the essence. Where a relationship is strong, each can support the other's emotional needs; but, where the relationship is weak, where there is lack of communication, where one partner abdicates his or her responsibility, there can be outbursts of anger and conflict between the parents.

Children, too, can get caught up in the conflict, with one or both of the parents or with each other. The phenomenon of sibling rivalry and problems of sibling relationships exist in every family, but the presence of a handicapped child can intensify these problems. Parents can become so absorbed in the care and attention of the special child that the interests, joys, and problems of the other children can become relegated to second place. For example, if a teenage child wants to have friends over to the house, will he react with embarrassment? Or again, older children in the family may resort to infantile behavior to get their parents' attention. The opposite may happen, as well. Children may become so motherly and overprotective that they will act much more grown-up than what would ordinarily be expected for their age.

The pressures on the family unit may become so severe that what began as only resentment toward the child's handicap may turn into resentment toward the child itself.

Two emotional factors that can be severely damaging are denial and overprotection. Parents who need to deny (beyond a reasonable time) their child's limitations will put unrealistic expectations on the child, resulting in a damaged parent-child relationship and causing serious emotional disturbances for the child. The other extreme would be to become so overprotective of the child that the child's true realistic potential could be stifled.

Some parents find it hard to discipline a handicapped child, possibly due to unresolved feelings of guilt. They may rationalize that the child should be allowed to do whatever he wants to do because he has so much more to learn and cope with. However, many brain-injured children respond well if they know what is expected of them.

Stage 3

The picture I have painted of this second stage of research and reintegration may appear hopelessly bleak. Maybe if the parents had to face all these problems and emotional adjustments alone, the prospects of reaching the final stage of recovery and mature adaptation would indeed be bleak. But the age is behind us when handicapped children would be shunted to the family closet and the door slammed. Community agencies are available to help support families in their tasks of helping handicapped children achieve their fullest potential. Two of the many invaluable services they render is to put families in touch with other families who have the same problems and to steer the family towards family counseling services.

THE HELPING PROFESSIONS

The final section of this chapter, hopefully, will be the most practical — what those in the helping professions can do to help parents along the road to mature adaptation. Since most chaplains, doctors, and nurses have contact with parents during the initial stage of shock and disorganization, I shall limit my comments to this first stage.

First of all, it is absolutely essential that we examine our own values regarding life and respect for life. For example, can we ourselves accept this deformed child as human, having value in himself or herself, precious in God's sight? Can we look at this child without revulsion? If we cannot, we can never communicate our loving concern to the parents. Parents will watch the facial expression of nurses and other personnel to detect feelings of revulsion. Maybe we do not give them a chance to see our faces; maybe we conveniently withdraw. As products of our environment, we also place a high premium on looks and body image. We may feel helpless and angry and anxious, and because we don't know what to say, we may communicate to the parents that we are not interested.

Obviously, if we are to help, we must be present to the parents. Our presence must be a loving one, in that it provides an atmosphere of acceptance, both of the parents and of their feelings of shock, disappointment, grief, anger. We must give the parents an opportunity to express all their feelings, while accepting unconditionally their worth as persons. Personally, I find it most trying to accept parents' feelings of anger. We must constantly remind ourselves that the anger directed toward us is not personal. The parents are feeling immeasurable pain and directing that pain and disillusionment and disappointment to the nearest object. A chaplain is often the object of anger insofar as he represents God to the parents. "What kind of God is *your* God anyway, to do such a thing?" The first thing *not* to do is try to defend God, as strong as the temptation is. As Elizabeth Kubler-Ross says, "Don't feel you have to defend God. He is big enough to take care of Himself."

Sometimes silence is the most appropriate response, especially when we don't know what to say or when nothing we can say is truly meaningful. A comforting touch of the hand, an arm around the parent, a shoulder to cry on — sometimes these nonverbal expressions communicate acceptance and understanding better than a thousand words. Also, this is no time to enter into the theology or philosophy of pain, suffering, or evil in the world. The parents do not need this now. Communicate to them that you feel their pain even though you don't know completely what they're going through.

When parents express guilt feelings about real or imagined wrongdoings, I try to reassure them that God is beyond the pettiness of meting out punishment upon innocent victims for the sins of others. If there is real guilt, sacramental confession may be in order somewhere down the line. The ultimate answer to guilt is that we don't know. We must be able to accept these guilt feelings without judging. I try to reassure parents that even if they have done something in their past, that they are responsible only for the present in their relationship with God. God forgives and forgets, but we sometimes find it much harder to forgive ourselves.

What do we say when parents ask in effect, "What's wrong with me as a propagator?" A consultant in genetics may help. Indeed, he may indicate that a definable hereditary basis exists for this anomaly. Usually, when this is true, both members of the couple carry what is called a recessive genetic trait which results in this tragedy. In any case, blame in any ordinary sense would be terribly wrong and misdirected. The parents must learn to accept this anomaly not as evidence of a shameful trait in one of them, but simply on the basis of an accident in development. In the vast majority of cases (perhaps in no case), no real blame can be directed against either parent.

The physician will probably also feel he should rely on the genetics expert to answer the question, "What is the likelihood of a similar abnormality in the next child?" It is important to realize that no attempt should be made to give guidance in an area which more properly belongs to a psychiatrist, physician, psychologist, or some other professional working with the parents.

When the question "Why?" is asked, probably the best answer in most cases is, "I don't know." Although more and more is being learned about congenital anomalies, I suspect that it still is rare for a physician to arrive at a specific and satisfactory answer in specific instances. Unless there is a specific answer, I find it best to attribute the defect to an accident of nature. We live in an imperfect world and things don't always work out the way we want them to. It is amazing that congenital defects do not occur more often, considering the intricate details of conception and fetal development.

A mother will feel supported if we help her realize that her feelings are natural. An attitude of warmth and acceptance is the most important attitude we can convey. This attitude is best communicated through actions rather than words.

It is also important to realize that parents need silence and to be alone at times, and that this is not to be equated with rejection of the child. We should also beware of making overly optimistic statements regarding the future or the child's potential. This kind of reassurance only serves to relieve tension in ourselves. Empathy, understanding, and patience are probably the three most important virtues to have in helping parents pass from the first stage to the second.

Although this chapter has attempted to present some psychological-emotional reactions of parents and siblings to the birth of a child with congenital anomalies, it would be false and an oversimplification to categorize all parents as having to go through the three stages described above. To try to neatly categorize the emotions of all parents of children with congenital anomalies would only be a projection of my own personal inadequacy in trying to give constructive counseling. I think a valid point of counseling is always to meet the client where he or she is.

In fact, the three stages I have presented are not nearly so neat or well-defined in practice. Many parents do not proceed rapidly through these stages, but can come stranded on the rocks of their emotional trauma. Often, they need to be reassured when they become angry or wonder if it's all worth it, and this can happen even after they have come to the stage of mature adaptation.

The extent to which any child reaches maximum potential depends on three factors: 1) The child's potential; 2) the quality of care, instruction, and guidance he receives; and 3) his own motivation or personal response, cooperation and effort. However, a handicapped child's feelings about himself and his handicap are primarily determined by the feelings and attitudes of his parents, family members, and others around him. The basis for his progress is established to a large degree in his home environment. The correct conclusion then is that the emotional climate in which the handicapped child lives is probably the most important factor in his life. On this point, I would like to quote Susanne Kohut:

> It is gratifying to see the many families who make a mature adaptation and who, through the process of adjustment, gain strength for themselves and can and do experience many satisfactions. The satisfactions derive from having successfully come to grips with the problems presented and from accepting the child, despite his limitations.

> Providing the child with parental love, making available to him the necessary physical and medical care; helping him to utilize social and educational opportunities; interpreting the child's needs and potentialities to his brothers and sisters, relatives, friends and neighbors; strengthening his ability to surmount everyday problems and crisis situations; enabling him to cope with the reactions of others and giving him understanding of his feelings to these reactions; and lastly fulfilling their responsibilities as parents as part of their faith in God, are some of the many wellsprings of justified pride and satisfaction for the parents and family members of the special child.

> A child is a delicate being, sensitive to the slightest wounds of fear, intolerance and thoughtlessness. His growth and development is affected by all who come in contact with him. The understanding professional person will wish to help those persons close to the child to enable him to receive the love, security, and understanding to weather the storm of his life-long injury and pain.[8]

FOOTNOTES:

1. E. E. Jacobs, "Troubled Parents — Their Feeling Toward the Handicapped," *Pastoral Psychology*, June 1965, pp. 36-40.

2. *Ibid.*

3. Susanne A. Kohut, "The Abnormal Child: His Impact on the Family," *Journal of the American Physical Therapy Association*, February 1966, Vol. 46, No. 2, p. 161.

4. *Ibid.*, p. 162.

5. Park J. White, "Helping Parents of Congenitally Malformed Children," *Religion & Health*, Sept. 1952, p. 26.

6. Kohut, *op. cit.*, p. 162.

7. Mary Marguerite Matheny, "Antidotes for Confusion," *The Crippled Child*, August 1957, pp. 11-12.

8. Kohut, *op. cit.*, p. 167.

Emotional Reactions in the Cancer Patient

SISTER VALERIA BRUNGARDT, CSA

When a patient learns that he has cancer, he and his family often undergo a severe psychological shock. Although the cancer patient may experience the same emotional stages as do patients with other illnesses, there is a difference. The implied meaning attached to the disease — pain, disfigurement, hospitalization, inability to care for one's family, disability, and possible death —trigger a series of intense emotional reactions.

Clinical psychologists who have studied the reactions of cancer patients identify four emotional responses evidenced in all patients. These include denial, anxiety, depression, and dependency, and they may appear singly or in combination. The degree to which these responses are manifested and the extent of counter-responses to cope with them vary with each individual. Some exaggerate these emotions and needs to a pathological degree, while others merely use them as expressions of severe stress with which the patient copes successfully.

Denial can be either conscious or unconscious. For example, the patient may recognize the nature of cancer but refuse to consider any outcome but an overly optimistic one. Or he can refuse to be concerned. He can accomplish this either through religious beliefs, by avoiding thinking about the situation, or by an apathetic response. A third form of denial refuses to consider the situation as threatening to the individual.

Those involved in caring for the cancer patient should encourage the patient to use denial in adaptive ways and discourage its use as a maladaptive means of meeting the threat of the illness. It is normal for a patient, upon first learning of the diagnosis of cancer, to be shocked and disbelieving and sometimes even apathetic. At this time, the chaplain can be available to listen, not in an attempt to support the patient's denial, but to allow him to cope with the situation in this way at the present time.

The removal of a malignant tumor often necessitates radical or disfiguring surgery, and the normal reaction to stress and threat is anxiety. Anxiety can be brought on by many things, including threat to life, health, or body integrity; exposure and embarrassment; pain; fatigue; change in diet; deprivation of sexual satisfaction; restriction of movement; interruption or loss of one's means of livelihood; precipitation of financial crises; rejection or ridicule from others as a result of condition; frustration of goals and expectations; confusion and uncertainty about the present and future; and separation from family and friends. The patient experiencing anxiety may feel uneasy and apprehensive. Feelings of helplessness and inadequacy may be present along with a sense of alienation and insecurity. The intensity of these feelings can range from mild to severe, sometimes severe enough to cause panic. The intensity of these feelings may be increased or diminished by interpersonal means.

Anxiety may significantly enhance the patient's discomfort, which he will subsequently interpret as increased pain. The patient may also construe anxiety as tension, nervousness, apprehension, or fear. Some patients may even deny the presence of anxiety, because they regard it as unmanly, or immature, or a sign of weakness. The patient's realistic interpretation of his plight and his anxious responses to it, is aided by the empathic concern of the doctor, nurse, and chaplain, which provides understanding, support, and security.

Another anticipated emotional response to cancer is depression. This response may be mild and transitory, but when it is strong, it often involves added symptoms of guilt and self-deprecation. This feeling of depression includes a negative outlook toward oneself, family members, hospital staff, and the world in general.

Each person has a unique concept of his body image, a useful fact to remember when attempting to understand the many complex reactions of people to changes in their health status. Body image may be considered the total, constantly changing and evolving perception of one's physical self as separate and distinct from others. This perception is based on inner sensations and functionings, as well as information derived from the external environment. Society also prescribes norms of physical appearance and behavior.

The perception of body image operates on both the conscious and unconscious levels. Thus, any alteration of this concept has important emotional ramifications, including feelings of increased dependency and low self-worth. Guilt feelings are often involved in depression, as though the individual is anticipating punishment for earlier wrongdoing. The patient's concern over expressed or unexpressed anger toward the persons closest to him may create guilt. This can set up a vicious circle of dependency, leading to anger, which leads to guilt, which fosters further dependency.

Most cancer patients experience guilt feelings which may interfere with treatment. The opportunity to openly discuss these guilt feelings can be helpful. Despite actual disability, much of this guilt is exaggerated and unrealistic, based on a fear of further bodily damage and pain. The total depression syndrome can be helped when the physician, nurse, and chaplain are aware of it and act in a supportive, empathic manner toward the patient and his family.

The fourth usual response to cancer is dependency. Cancer, with its extensive diagnostic testing, therapeutic procedures, and hospitalization, forces the patient to be dependent upon hospital personnel and the doctor. Initial denial of dependency with an attempt to maintain status quo relationships, needs, and emotions is commonly seen. However, as disability increases, dealing with dependency in this manner proves ineffective. When a patient loses his independence, he may regress to a childlike role of helplessness and display great need for care. A person who has been dependent throughout his entire life thrives on added dependency; his insatiable dependency needs lead to anticipation of receiving further care from family, physician, and nursing staff. If the family of the patient or others are unable to meet these extensive dependency needs, he will often become irritable, hostile, or angry. When this happens, a great deal of skill in handling the cancer patient is required. The patient must be helped to maintain his motivation for life, health, and productivity.

Since many patients associate cancer with a lingering painful death, the question often arises as to whether or not the patient should be told that he has cancer. Most patients are reasonably emotionally healthy individuals, and they want and need to know. They have things to do, plans to make, and unfinished business to attend. The human organism has built-in mechanisms for dealing with painful reality.

Because man is a rational being, he tries to make sense out of his environment. If well-meaning people try to keep the facts from him, he is likely to fill in the gap with something conjured up from his imagination. Often, it is more frightening than the truth and puts the patient into a worse state. In addition, if the patient is not told about his condition, his family is forced to carry a double burden — coping with their own reactions and feelings and simultaneously trying to keep up appearances for the patient. Therefore, if the patient possesses the inner resources to cope with the news (and most patients do), he should be told the diagnosis.

When told of his illness, the patient may react in various ways; he may cry, become hysterical, angry, depressed, or withdrawn. Those responsible for breaking the news should remember that honesty is not equivalent to unvarnished truth without emotional support. Hope can and must be given in the context of the reality of the illness.

On the other hand, the patient might react by calling upon his inner resources and experiencing a higher level of emotion functioning than before. Some patients who learn they have cancer discover unusual strength and spiritual resources. These people command admiration and respect. They also avail themselves of the opportunity to talk with others, such as their families, doctors, nurses, and chaplains, when they need strength and help. Consequently, we must not avoid the patient's questions and concerns. Rather, we must allow him to express his thoughts and feelings without interruption and listen and respond helpfully. And we must remember that it is not always necessary to have an answer to the patient's question as long as we help him find the answer or refer him to a person who will have it.

With current medical knowledge and skills, many cancer patients reach the stage of palliative care. Palliative measures may include radiotherapy, chemotherapy, or home care. In considering palliative care, it is important to treat the patient as a person with an illness rather than as a problem of palliative care. Rather than speaking of a cure, those responsible for the patient's care should say that the cell growth has been slowed or stopped. A hopeful but realistic attitude will result in a more useful psychological environment for the patient. Incurability is a state of the body; hopelessness is a state of the mind and should be avoided at all cost. Whether the patient adapts to his illness sooner or later or never depends a great deal on the patient himself and his personality. The patient's response to his illness and therapy will have a substantial effect on palliative therapy.

During and after radiation or chemotherapy, the patient may react to his condition through hypochondria, paranoia, and obsessive-compulsive reactions. These reactions must be dealt with if the patient is to become rehabilitated and resume his place in his family and in the community with minimum stress. If the patient exhibits hypochon-driacal tendencies, he should be encouraged to return to work if possible and resume his usual home life and recreations. Establishing and maintaining satisfactory relations with other people will help dispel paranoia, and help the patient feel significant and worthwhile. Perhaps there is no other disease that is such a threat to "wholeness" as cancer, and adequate understanding and empathy for "what the patient is going through" can contribute much to the patient's rehabilitation.

Neither x-ray nor cobalt therapy cause pain or discomfort during the time of the treatment, but skin changes such as reddening may result after several days of treatment, and such changes can pose a threat to the body image. Depending upon the area of the body being treated, the patient may also experience nausea, vomiting, or diarrhea. Radiation sickness can be influenced by the emotional state of the patient, so he should be reassured that these side-effects are normal. A program of rest and diversion in pleasant surroundings is of great help to the patient at this time.

What does death mean to a patient? Certainly, the concept involves feelings of fear, loneliness, and abandonment in many patients. Abandonment is a particular fear of many patients with terminal illness. Patients experiencing such feelings receive untold help and comfort from someone who merely spends time with them. Needless to say, if one is sure of his own feelings and has a sound philosophy, the exact words he uses when speaking to the patient do not matter; his manner, tone of voice, expression on the face, and empathy for the patient are all that matter.

Probably the most effective antidote to fear of death is the will to live. The patient with advanced cancer is faced with the stark reality that he has a limited life span, but often this awareness stimulates him to unbelievable courage, strength, and insights. The emotionally healthy person, rather than concentrating on the fact that his life expectancy is limited, will often say, "Thank God, I have one more year to live."

When the patient's expected life span is longer, some want nothing more than to forget their surgery and palliative treatments. Those in the helping professions can assist the patient by encouraging and supporting him and by understanding and accepting the patient's feelings. Emotional support can help foster the patient's sense of dignity and actually lessen his experience of pain. Helping the patient resume responsibility and decision-making increases his sense of self-control and self-esteem.

Dying with "dignity" requires a feeling of personal self-worth and of control of the immediate environment, limited though it may be. Such "dignity" is more easily achieved in a home setting, and home support should definitely be considered. Ongoing work with the family to facilitate the grief process may help prevent future medical and psychiatric disease. Such grief work should be considered part of the family care.

In closing, I might add that the intimate association with life and death and the stages in between arouse conscious and unconscious fears of our own vulnerability. Recognition of this fact is important as are our all-out efforts on the patient's behalf. Hopefully, we should always be able to say, "I did all that was possible."

The Psychological Effects of Colostomy and Ileostomy

SISTER JUDITH SCHUBERT, SM, BA

A total colectomy is the complete removal of the colon and often the rectum as well; therefore the surgical procedure produces an artificial means of defecation. This artificial means is created by producing an ileostomy or a colostomy. An ileostomy is formed by bringing an end of the small intestine through the abdominal wall to serve as an opening for the intestines. Here the discharged contents are unformed and cannot be regulated; therefore some type of dressing must be continually worn over the stoma. On the other hand, a colostomy is formed by bringing an end of the large intestine through the abdominal wall to serve as an opening. Here the contents are more formed.

Two main reasons for performing this kind of surgery are bowel cancer and ulcerative colitis. It is important to keep in mind the difference in causes between the two operations: The former is physical in cause, while the latter is emotional. Until recently, many psychiatrists had reservations about suggesting this operation to patients with psychosomatic illnesses (e.g., ulcerative colitis), because they subscribed to the theory that if the psychosomatic target organ was removed, the illness would appear somewhere else since the conflict had not yet been resolved. This theory has lately been challenged.

In brief, the surgery for such illnesses involves three basic steps: 1) Removal of an organ; 2) closure of the anus; and 3) creation of an artificial orifice. This procedure, which permanently alters bowel function and control, can cause great trauma in the patient. Such control is learned very early in life and, in western society, is surrounded by highly charged emotional associations.

The presence of a stoma does not preclude living a full, productive, and quite active life. Often, the problem lies in popular misconceptions as well as the emotional fears of the patient. The location of the stoma is selected so as not to interfere with a waistline, skin folds, other scars, etc. It usually protrudes approximately one inch, especially in the cases of urinary stomas and ileostomies, to allow the liquids to be effectively managed.

Patients with colectomies have varied physiological problems depending upon the structure or type of surgery that is performed. To identify such needs it is helpful to distinguish between the different types of surgical procedures. They include the following:

1.   Ileal conduit   A surgical procedure in which the urine is excreted from a passage produced from a piece of the small intestine.

2.   Ileostomy   A stoma produced through some piece of the small intestine.

3.   Colstomy
     a. Sigmoid   A stoma produced through the lower portion of the large intestine.

     b. Transverse   A stoma produced through the upper portion of the large intestine.

A classic study on this topic, done by Sutherland[1] in 1952, identified four major areas of patient concern: Social, work, family, and sexual activity. A follow-up study, conducted by Orbach and Talbent in 1964, identified feelings and physical needs which were common to persons with an ostomy as long as five to 15 years after the operation. "The feelings were depression, altered perception of the person's own body, and a lowered self-esteem."[2] It is apparent, then, that even after a long span of years some patients still experience feelings of loss and grief, loss because of body mutilation and grief because of worry. It is very important, therefore, to keep patients physically dry, clean, and odor-free so that they do not feel like outcasts.

In terms of physical management, the various types of help sought include: 1) Learning self care; 2) avoiding skin break-outs, odor, gas; and 3) managing the stoma, its techniques, its appliances. Periodically, the chosen appliance may not be properly adjusted, allowing leakage to occur. For the patient's sake, it is essential to correct this disfunction at the earliest moment. Common skin problems such as ulcerations, eruptions from irritations, etc., can also be cured fairly simply. Sexual functions need not be inhibited due to this type of surgery. Generally speaking, the operation does not prohibit most normal human functions. The real challenge lies not in physically but in psychologically coping with this procedure.

One of the most devastating emotional factors prohibiting recovery for the patient is fear: Fear of being considered a "leper," fear of spillage, fear of odor, fear of being incomplete and unacceptable to others. Historically one of man's earliest achievements is bowel control. Today, especially in the western world, lack of control implies a return to infancy and subsequent loss of self-esteem. A stoma therefore is unacceptable to everyone, medical personnel included, because the concept is associated with a sense of inadequacy and dirtiness.

In this area of fear, one of the initial challenges the patient must face following surgery is the visible results of the operation. Many patients feel emotionally unprepared for the surgery and therefore experience great shock in first confronting the stoma. Even when the patient is well-prepared, the first sight of the ostomy is always upsetting. Women periodically become more shattered as a result of the operation because the image of a perfect body becomes hopelessly unattainable. The body has been literally mutilated. "In the stoma patient, there is not just a scar; an opening has been created from which wastes flow, uncontrolled, and these, instead of falling unseen into the toilet, she must touch with her hands."[3] Consequently, depression in the postoperative stage is common and understandable since the body has been radically changed and self-esteem may be fluctuating or lost.

No event is more dreaded by the ostomy patient than spillage. When it happens, an overwhelming sense of shame often overtakes the patient. Since this occurrence cannot always be completely controlled, some patients tend to live in isolation. Profound feelings of self-deprecation may not only be associated with spillage but may represent an abiding attitude toward themselves.

Another reason for a retreat from social groups is the unexpected expulsion of gas. Aside from being uncontrollable, ostomy odor depends upon what food is eaten as well as what oral medicine is taken. Since the patient fears embarrassment in public society, he may avoid even the possibility of such an occurrence by isolating himself from the social milieu.

If, in the postoperative period, major emotional concerns of the patient are not discussed, he may remain uninformed, afraid, and the victim of myths. Among the greatest myths are those pertaining to sexual matters. Sexual adjustments are very possible the more the patient is informed. In the male the question of impotency is often the main concern, but the myth that the operation will disturb the patient's potency is unfounded. The female's fear of being ugly and incomplete often leaves her repulsed by sexual activity. "Every patient's self-image is altered by this surgery. His capacity to rebuild or reestablish a workable self-image is intimately related to a healthy social response and even more closely related to his capacity to respond sexually."[4] If sex is an intimate type of communication of love and affection for the patient, he will need to have a deep caring and love displayed toward him at this traumatic time. More than others, patients with mutilative surgery need to be encouraged, supported, and deeply loved if they are to function normally.

In a research and demonstration project prepared by the Office of Vocational Rehabilitation, a questionnaire was sent to over 1400 persons with an ileostomy. The results of the study indicated that 85 percent of the patients were in very good physical health, whereas previous to their operations, half of them were chronic invalids. At the same time, most of the patients lacked emotional peace of mind, indicating that physical success did not counteract feelings of personal inadequacy. In general, men were much more preoccupied and resentful of their illness than women.

Within marital relationships the issue of sexual functioning remained a key psychological issue. The spouse's reaction to the patient's illness is essential for positive or negative sexual abilities of the patient. For example, the men usually relied on their wives for nursing during the postoperative period; consequently, "the husband's perception of his wife, and whether she was a person who accepted the sight and smell of his wound and stoma in the immediate postoperative period was most important."[5] The survey indicated that wives often became embarrassed over their husbands because of reduced income, lack of social activities, and the ugliness of the stoma which they viewed.

On the other hand, male spouses tended to take their wives' illness more in stride. Despite this, women had a deeper fear of not being acceptable to their spouses. "The marital relationship of any colostomy patient was a powerful force for good or evil, and the spouse was often the key to the patient's eventual success or failure in adapting to his disability."[6] In order to encourage the future adaptive patterns of the patient, family members generally need professional assistance in understanding the psychological challenges of the illness.

As has been mentioned, some of the adaptive problems of patients with these types of operations include severe humiliation over any accident involving spillage, concern over noise due to gas, fear of injury to the stoma. Such preoccupations often reduce the patient to a hypochondriac state. Therefore, the most primary psychological treatment involves these issues of personal concern. In order to deal with them effectively, every stoma patient needs to express negative feelings, fears, doubts, and anxieties. All team members must be aware of the many emotional difficulties and challenges that are part of the patient's experience. Since, in this operation, the cure often seems worse than the complaint, team members and family must be willing to listen and to support the patient in his process of "coping." Often it is helpful to encourage participation in ostomy clubs. In recent surveys, most patients agreed that other patients who had gone through similar surgeries were the most helpful to them.

In conclusion, building interpersonal relationships, readapting to society, and overcoming fears remain three of the most important emotional concerns of the patient. The family and team members play a vital role in this healing process of readjustment. It is essential to emphasize rehabilitation for the ostomy patient, not just concentrate on the physical stoma. A colectomy is performed for the purpose of living. Keeping this fact in mind will help the patient adapt to a fuller and richer future life.

FOOTNOTES:

1. A. Sutherland, "The Psychological Impact of Cancer and Cancer Surgery," *Cancer*, Vol. 5, No. 5, Sept. 1952, pp. 857-872.

2. Ann Gallagher, "Body Image Changes in the Patient With a Colostomy," *The Nursing Clinics of North America*, December 1972, p. 670.

3. Edith Lenneberg and Norman Sohn, "Modern Concepts in the Management of Patients With Intestinal and Urinary Stomas," *Clinical Obstetrics and Gynecology*, June 1972, p. 565.

4. B. Dlin, A. Perman, and E. Ringold, "Psychosexual Response to Ileostomy and Colostomy," *The American Journal of Psychiatry*, Sept. 1969, p. 380.

5. R. Druss and J. O'Connor, "Psychologic Response to Colostomy," *General Psychiatry*, January 1968, p. 54.

6. *Ibid.*

The Stroke Patient

SISTER CARMEL MEYER, CSA, PhD, MA

In my interest and concern for stroke patients, I recently contacted the American Rehabilitation Center in Minneapolis to find out what material was available for a person in the Pastoral Care Department who was interested in doing more effective work for those who had suffered a cerebrovascular stroke. The answer I received was totally expected: "We have nothing. In fact, a speaker here recently made the statement that scarcely no one is available among chaplains, nuns or laymen who is psychologically or emotionally geared to help a stroke patient. Few are even aware of the silent cries for help from a stroke patient."

In 1967, there were over 2,000,000 stroke patients in the country, 200,000 of whom died.[1] If cardiovascular patients are to be rehabilitated, not only should the occupational therapy department be involved, but also the pastoral care department. Because of the nature of this department, those who function in it ought to be highly sensitive to and deeply aware of human suffering, even when it can be expressed only through pain-filled eyes that gaze hopelessly on a world that seems to have closed its door on all that makes life worth living.

Perhaps it is understandable why some doctors and nurses hate to see CVA's admitted to the hospital and why they want them moved to a nursing home quickly. Because doctors and nurses think in terms of health, life, activity, the stroke patient seems to be medically uninteresting because he fails to display any of the three mentioned above. But for the chaplain or his counterpart, ministering the stroke patient can be a rewarding experience.

Strokes vary from mild to very severe. Patients with milder afflictions have more confidence and more hope, feeling that good health is just around the corner. This kind of patient must make use of those measures that will keep him from a recurring stroke of greater magnitude, such as avoiding harmful foods, avoiding pressure, getting adequate rest, etc. If the doctor fails to take time to talk to the patient along these lines, the chaplain may prove to be a support to him.

In various degrees, stroke patients suffer from sensory loss. Extreme cases can glibly be labeled "vegetables," a term not only vulgar in its use but hopeless in its connotation. The brain never stops its activity, anymore than the heart. "Although the brain is only a bit more than 1/50 of a man's body, it receives about 1/6 of the blood pumped out by the heart and consumes 1/5 of the entire oxygen supply."[2] Since this is true, great hope needs to be generated, especially by doctors, nurses, chaplains, media people, etc.

Too often, the stroke patient is treated almost as if he is an object not a patient. He finds himself in a hospital bed before he knows it, having suffered a neurological disorder, to say nothing of the depression that is awaiting him. Often, he can understand more than is realized, even though he does not and cannot give a suitable response. Therefore, it is unwise to talk as if he were not there, or as if he cannot hear or understand. In a personal account, Douglas Ritchie tells how annoyed he was with the doctor who spoke to others in a normal tone in his presence, but spoke loudly to him as if to a dull foreigner. But he was irritated most of all by the well-intentioned nurse who spoke baby talk to him.[3]

Patients who cannot understand words may yet derive comfort from the way in which a visitor speaks the words. A great deal of nonverbal communication passes from one to another — the set of the head, the expressive face and eyes, the posture of the body. Patients may respond even though they cannot fully comprehend the words.[4] When speaking to a stroke patient, the speaker should talk to him and treat him as an adult, even though he may act childish. Nouns should be used in preference to adjectives or other parts of speech. Carmen McBride, in her book *Silent Victory*, tells how her husband could understand nouns, but not conjunctions and prepositions.[5]

Dr. McKenzie Buck who writes about his own stroke advises use of simple vocabulary, with short phrases. He asked his wife to keep a careful log of all his reactions and activities. "In two years, I accurately recalled all major events and conversations with complete absence of assistance from those around me."[6]

It is generally admitted that professional personnel too often monopolize conversations, thus depriving the patient of the opportunity to vent his detrimental self-concern. Conversely, opportunity for free expression may ward off pre-psychotic depression.

Dr. Buck also maintains that the stroke patient need not lose his remaining verbal abilities, if he is constantly verbally stimulated by participating in pleasurable communicative experiences. "This non-direct interpersonal activity is far more valuable than any regulated remedial drills — especially in initial stages." The patient is aided by attentive and nondirective listeners, and often a pleasant facial expression may not accurately reflect his true emotional state.[7]

A stroke patient who is deprived of speech (aphasia) or who is paralyzed on one side of his body (hemiplegia) must learn to spell, write, and walk anew. He faces personality conflicts, over and above the physical handicap. At times irrational behavior, unaccountable anger, throwing of objects within reach, and deliberately hurting the ones he loves most are all related to his illness. At times he suffers from severe depression, resentment, and bitterness. He may use language he doesn't want to use — swearing, cursing, four-letter words. Great understanding and patience is required at this time. It is necessary to remember that the stroke patient's condition is unique. The cancer patient and the heart patient live or die with their faculties reasonably intact; the stroke patient generally lives, but in a world which has suddenly collapsed. Is it any wonder then that crying characterizes the stroke patient, a helpless physical demonstration over which he has no control.[8]

Besides a possible change in personality, the body image of the stroke patient undergoes a severe change. Before the stroke he may have been a dynamic, vigorous, successful person, admired by his associates; now he cannot speak, write, or walk. Considering how our American culture stresses the body beautiful syndrome, the stroke patient's whole value system must be explored. Body image values are good when present, but their absence can be extremely disturbing.

Every chaplain and counselor is in a position to help a disabled stroke patient progress toward better psychological adjustment. Although the patient's speech or use of disabled limbs may never return, his self-image must. When God made him, He made him in His own Image, and no stroke or other influence can rob him of this reality.

One of the most important factors in aiding the stroke patient to return to normalcy is his spouse and family. If spouse and family evidence love and maturity, much is already resolved. However, consider the case of the wife who lets her husband do everything, who is the clinging type, the over-enamored admirer of masculine strength and virility. What will a stroke do to this kind of person. It can shatter her. If she is in the menopause period, the consequences can be even more severe. Often her sexual life suffers.

Since speaking to her physician is out of the question, usually the pastor can often offer the necessary guidance. She may confide in him her frustrations and her fears, and he then has the opportunity to point out her hidden strengths, which can be instrumental in contributing to her husband's recovery. Her attitude, too, will affect the whole family, because often they will take their cue from her. Thus, an understanding and knowledgeable pastor can truly help her, the family, and, thereby, the patient. Acceptance by the family is crucial for the stroke patient. The minister can be a key to easing a difficult readjustment. When has a sense of love, of caring, and of real concern failed in its impact?

Finally, heroes are still invaluable sources of inspiration. For example, Walt Whitman suffered a stroke at 39, followed by many other strokes, and still wrote *Leaves of Grass*. Louis Pasteur performed some of his finest work after he had a stroke at the age of 45. At the time of his death, examination disclosed extensive deterioration in one hemisphere of his brain. Handel wrote perhaps his most magnificent musical work, *Messiah*, after he had a stroke. And there are countless others whose handicap proved greatness. Therefore, let us not underestimate the ability of the stroke patient to survive or our ability to help him.

FOOTNOTES:

1. Irene Ramey, "The Stroke Patient is Interesting," *Forum*, Vol. VI, No. 3, 1967, p. 272.

2. S. H. Page, et. al., *Strokes: How They Occur and What Can Be Done*, E. P. Dutton and Co., New York City, 1961, p. 32.

3. Frederick Al Whitehouse, "Stroke," *American Journal of Nursing*, Oct. 1963, pp. 81-87.

4. *Ibid.*

5. Carmen McBride, *Silent Victory*, Nelson-Hall Co., Chicago, 1969, p. 28.

6. McKenzie Buck, "Adjustments During Recovery From Stroke," *American Journal of Nursing*, Vol. 64, No. 10, pp. 93-95.

7. *Ibid.*

8. Montague Ullman, "Disorders of Body Image After Stroke," *American Journal of Nursing*, Oct. 1964, pp. 89-91.

Ministry to Persons with Physical Disabilities

PEGGY PFAB, BA

"The greatest service the pastor can offer the disabled is to walk with him through the valley of anguish, depression, and anger; to stand at his side in the struggle with confusions and doubts; to work with him toward a new inner balance, as well as toward a realistic acceptance and accommodation of what the future will hold for him, and to do all of this in the spirit and as the representative of the community of the faithful."[1]

The quotation above represents one person's conception of how to minister to a person with a physical disability. They are beautiful and moving words, containing a profound insight, but they pose a real and difficult challenge to anyone who wants to function as a minister to persons with disabilities. This is a challenge that I, personally, have become really aware of only in the last couple of years. Currently, I am teaching adults, all of whom have quite severe physical disabilities and some of whom are also mentally retarded. Consequently, I have encountered some of the special problems of working with persons with disabilities, as well as some of the special rewards. This chapter attempts to present some ideas I have gained as a result both of my experience in this field and from my reading on the subject. The emphasis will be on the services the minister can offer to persons having disabilities, and the focus will be on persons with physical disabilities, rather than mental or emotional.

In trying to gain some insight into the area, I will first of all give a general definition of the term physical disability. Then I will deal briefly with some of the stereotypes that society imposes on people with physical disabilities; stereotypes that are detrimental to the growth and development of persons. Then I will take a look at what research has found to be some general concerns of persons with disabilities, and what special ways ministers can best relate to those needs; then a brief look at some of the questions the minister must personally deal with to become more effective in this situation.

Often the words "disability" and "handicap" are used interchangeably, yet Beatrice Wright, in her book on the psychological aspects of physical disability, cites a distinction between "disability" and "handicap." She defines disability as "a condition of impairment, physical or mental, having an objective aspect that can usually be described by a physician. . . . A handicap is the cumulative result of the obstacles which disability interposes between the individual and his maximum functional level."[2] A disability, then, refers to a medical reality, and a handicap refers to a relationship between the physical atttributes of a person and the environment. She defines this as the "somatopsychological relation . . . a relation dealing with these variations in physique that affect the psychological situation of a person by influencing the effectiveness of his body as a tool for actions or by serving as a stimulus for himself and others." The disability (a medical, objective reality) imposes certain limitations, and is a loss or a denial of something valuable, which affects the person's interrelationships with society.[3]

There are numerous medical causes of disabilities — spina bifida, hydrocephalus, vision or hearing loss, muscular dystrophy, epilepsy, cerebral palsy, brain injury syndrome, etc. All of these, of course, have different medical and physical bases and different symptoms, and thus each imposes different limitations upon the person. In addition, within any of these groupings, each individual person will experience different symptoms, limitations, and abilities. Consequently, making generalizations is both dangerous and erroneous. Yet, there are some general things that can be said about people experiencing physical disabilities that can be helpful and usually applicable.

Before examining those generalizations that are usually applicable to most disabled persons, let us first examine those inaccurate stereotypes imposed by society that do not have a sound basis in reality and that contribute to the depersonalization and devaluation of the individual. These generalizations must be dispelled before we can begin to minister effectively to individual persons who have disabilities. Following is a list and brief discussion of some of the commonly accepted myths concerning people with disabilities.

First: All persons with physical disabilities are handicapped persons. As Beatrice Wright states, not every person with a disability perceives it as a handicap, if the disability does not interfere significantly with the person's vocational, social, and psychological functioning.[4] The extent to which a person with a disability feels himself to be handicapped may be much less than the observer may assume.

Second: All persons with physical disabilities naturally experience more frustration, irritability, regression, restlessness, and other negative effects.[5] Wright cites many studies, the findings of which show that this is not necessarily true. Disabled people may either lower their goals in accordance with their abilities, or they meet frustration by substituting a goal that is attainable and therefore brings the same satisfaction.[6]

Third: People with disabilities are primarily more religious than the general populace. Indeed, many people may experience a stimulus to a greater spiritual growth as a result of a disability or especially a sudden onset of a disability. However, the evidence indicates that physical disability will not necessarily throw an individual into a search for life's ultimate meaning or for God or into a great encounter with the problem of theodicy. In fact, in sudden disabling experiences, the predisability personality pattern — in terms of the psychological, sociological, and spiritual dimensions —was very similar to the disability pattern.[7] In terms of the religious attitudes of persons with disabilities from birth, my own observations suggest that, as with most children's attitudes, the religious views and values of such persons would have more to do with the environment and the significant persons within the environment than with any specific influence of the disability on his religious attitudes.

Fourth: People with disabilities are more sensitive and profound, and have more understanding of life. Wright contends that this is not necessarily true. She maintains that "soul-searching" experiences are necessary for the attainment of depth and understanding, and, in that sense, the suffering involved in a disability may deepen the person's awareness and understanding. But she also points out that "soul-torturing" experiences — in which the individual feels overwhelmed and unable to find a way out of depression and despair —may lead to the opposite qualities of bitterness, callousness, resentment, etc. It is the process of adjusting to suffering that helps separate the trivial from the important and thus leads to a greater understanding and to more human values.[8]

Fifth: Persons with physical disabilities, especially persons with injured spinal cords, either do not or should not have sexual interests, desires, or the capacity for sexual relationships. This, in fact, is one of the major problem areas for people with disabilities. Dr. Cole, from the University of Minnesota Medical School Program on Human Sexuality, found in his questioning of many young men in wheelchairs that if they had a choice between walking again and normal sexual functioning, they would choose sexual functioning.[9]

Different sets of statistics are available, but most studies show that, with a sensitive and knowing partner, the vast majority of males can have erections. Fewer experience orgasm or are capable of intercourse, but, with sex counseling of both partners, recent studies are more optimistic. For women with spinal cord injuries, the menstrual cycle usually resumes within six months, and conception, pregnancy, and delivery can be quite normal — barring psychological obstacles.[10]

Treatment of sexual dysfunction in a spinal cord injured person must be primarily psychological. The patient must be able to discuss his or her sex life openly in order to get some honest answers and some realistic help with technique as well as attitudes.[11] In terms of attitudes, the same problems apply to people who have been disabled since birth — a real struggle in finding sexual identity and adjustment. Often, this struggle has more to do with unrealistic ideals of physique and the taboos of discussing sexuality imposed by society, than it has with actual physical inability. With openness, counseling, and experimentation, the majority of persons with physical disabilities can achieve some level of sexual gratification.

Sixth: Persons with severe disabilities will experience the most severe reactions and have the most difficulty in adjusting to the disability. In reality, often persons with milder disabilities tend to show greater conflict and difficulty in adjusting than persons with more severe disabilities.[12] Those with milder disabilities may retain longer the hope of being able to live a "normal" life, when they will never quite be able to do that. They may never realistically accept their limitations.[13]

Seventh: The person with a physical disability is also often mentally retarded or psychologically maladjusted, incapable of assuming responsibility for decision-making, or unable to cope with honesty and realism. Disabled persons, especially people who have cerebral palsy, particularly resent this misconception. Persons who are spastic, who cannot speak, and who may have some tendency to drool because of inability to control muscles, have indicated that people often assume that they are also deaf, retarded, or emotionally unstable.

Merely a brief look at some of the most common detrimental stereotypes imposed by society makes it obvious that an injustice is done when all individuals in a group are categorized as being a certain way. In fact, there is great diversity in personality structures, value systems, needs, and feelings among people with physical disabilities, just as there is among people in any other grouping. But bearing in mind the uniqueness of the individual and of his way of coping, we can identify some problems and adjustments that seem to be common to persons who experience physical disability. What we want to identify are the common questions and problems that present themselves to the person who is in the process of coping with a disability.

Among disabled persons, there is a distinction between those who experience a sudden disabling accident or disease and those who have been disabled from birth. Typically, even a gradual change in physique or ability to function is recognized, not gradually, but as a sudden, startling fact.[14] Even if the disability has been present from birth, there is a time when there comes a more sudden consciousness of it. Often, the full impact hits at puberty, when the adolescent realizes with sudden forcefulness that he or she will not outgrow the disability, and will have to go through life, being different from "normal" people.[15]

So, one of the common experiences is that, regardless of the type of disability, the age of onset, or the extent of the disability, there is a point at which the individual has to come to terms with what it means in his or her own life. Keeping in mind that this process is a fluid one, varying in length and intensity according to the individual, there are some common stages in the process of acceptance and coping.

Most authors liken this process to the process of mourning that takes place after the death of a loved one. In the case of a disability, the mourning is for the endeared state that was. There is often an inability or unwillingness to sever the ties with this prior state. The person often has extreme difficulty in recognizing other abilities and assets he still possesses because all of his attention is focused on the most obvious reality — the loss.

McEver, writing on the special problems in ministering to spinal cord injured persons, describes four main stages a person moves through in learning to cope with this disability. Although these are concerned specifically with spinal cord injured persons, they seem to be general enough to be helpful in considering the process that any person would go through in coping with a disability. These stages are: 1) Shock, 2) defensive retreat, 3) acknowledgment, and 4) adaptation.

The shock period is that period during which the first psychological realization of real danger or threat occurs. The person realizes his complete dependency. Often, he has no control over bladder or bowels or over movement. Perhaps he is unaware at this stage of the extent of the injury or disease. At this point, he experiences feelings of extreme helplessness and anxiety.[16]

In the stage of defensive retreat, there is a great deal of denial. The person reassures himself that the disability makes no real difference, or that it is only a temporary difference. This stage is often characterized by extreme anger, or by an autistic, wishful-thinking mentality. The fact that the person is often prevented from expressing this anger physically (by means of angry shouting, pacing, etc.) often increases his frustration to almost unbearable levels.

The next stage — acknowledgment — represents a new encounter with reality, an awareness on the part of the patient that he is no longer the way he was.[17] In the case of a disability from birth, it is an awareness that he is not, and never will be, like other people. This stage is one of self-deprecation, involving feelings of worthlessness and inferiority. It represents a period of grief and depression. Often the person can overcome these feelings by mobilizing his own natural inner resources. If this stage lasts too long or the depression becomes too overwhelming, it may become pathological. If this goes on for more than two to four months, the person may need some special help to enable him to move out of it. Two very real dangers associated with this particular stage is the development of a sense of either overdependence or underdependence.[18]

Once the person begins to realistically accept and deal with the situation he is in the final stage of adaptation. In this stage he recognizes his limitations, modifies his self-image, and finds a sense of worth and dignity that is based on an affirmation of self and the belief that life can still be enjoyable even though he may have to make some changes.[19]

It is at this point that the patient undergoes a change in self-identity and values. His value structure is enlarged to encompass those values that are still available to him and that enable him to live in the present with the belief that he has something to offer others, as well as the belief that life has something to offer him. At this point, values such as faith, brotherhood, etc., may take on new meaning.[20] Values directly related to physique and the ability to be active may undergo radical change. The person's value system may undergo a change, so that the more important values are those that are based more on the uniqueness of the person — the emotional and spiritual aspects of personhood — and on the importance of "being" over "doing." However, keep in mind the warning that appeared earlier in this chapter: The person does not *necessarily* develop this kind of value structure; it depends on many influences in the person and in the environment.

At this point the support, understanding, and respect of the people around him are very important, as is their sensitivity. It will greatly help if they have a sense of when to listen, when to be empathetic, when to confront. The most important thing to keep in mind is that the person needs to work through the problem himself, and that to deny him this opportunity is to deny him the healing process.[21]

Given the uniqueness of all individuals, including those with disabilities, and also some of the common problems that have to be faced in coming to terms with a disability, what can the minister offer to the person involved in this struggle? An effective helper, in the professional sense, must know the subject and also be able to do something with this knowledge.[22] The primary tool in a helping relationship is the person of the helper — his problem-solving ability, his values, beliefs, purposes, and perceptions. The most effective helper tends to be the kind of person who views events in a larger perspective, is self-revealing, involved, altruistic, process-oriented. He is a freeing person, to whom personal growth or "becoming" is a major concern.[23]

An important consideration when working with persons with

physical disabilities is an ability to work as a member of a helping team. Since one goal for the person with a disability is to learn to deal realistically with his environment, it is important for all members of the helping team to work together to facilitate this process. Thus, it is essential that the minister, as well as the other helping people in the environment, respond to the person in an honest, authentic, and compassionate way — recognizing and respecting the humanness and value of the person and the abilities he has.

Listening is an especially important function since speech may be made more difficult by the disability and many people in the environment may not have, or take, the time required to really listen. It is important to listen not only to what is said, but also to what is not said — the message between the words.[24] Participatory listening, in which the helper is involved, vulnerable, and honest, tells the person in a very real way that the helper sees him as valuable and important. This can have very deep ramifications; especially for the person who is still struggling with the problem of self-affirmation.

Listening, offering support, helping the person distinguish between realistic and unrealistic goals, helping his search for new meanings, examining values and determining which are his real values and which are values imposed by society, helping him to struggle with the problem of meaning and worth in his life — these are the tasks of the helping professions in regard to persons with physical disabilities.

Does the disabled person have any specific needs that are best served by a minister? Are there any special resources that the minister can bring to this situation? There are many. The minister's real area of service involves precisely such things as values, meanings, faith, and hope so often needed by the person trying to come to grips with a disability. The symbolism of the minister and of the Church — even when it is not explicitly verbalized — can often affirm the value of life and of humanness on a much more profound level than that of activities and physique. The traditional resources of the Church — prayer, Scripture reading, Sacraments — can be extremely comforting and encouraging when used at the appropriate time and in the appropriate setting.

Religion can help the person mobilize his own resources to confront the problem.[25] Thus, the perceptive minister can use his professional, theological perspective to help the person clarify and analyze where he is at, what his resources are, and how to put them to work. Since the person's religious values and ultimate concerns greatly influence the process of rehabilitation, the minister can help the patient determine where he is at in these areas. McEver describes three categories or patterns of religious ideas and values that might prove helpful in this process of clarification. They are: 1) A religion of works; 2) a religion of pleasure; 3) a religion of faith.[26]

Persons who subscribe to a religion of works are mainly concerned with activities, functions, "doing." A threat to such a person's physical functioning severely threatens his self-image. Sin and guilt are seen as a failure to live up to one's potentials. This person may consider death more desirable than a life of dependency. Grace may seem to be a foolish concept, since this person has a great difficulty in receiving.

The religion of pleasure sees life as good insofar as unpleasant experiences are avoided. Financial security, sexual fulfillment, and peace of mind are absolutized. This person may be unconcerned with self-improvement, since this might involve a great deal of pain. He may show signs of being overly dependent and unmotivated. For this person, suffering has no meaning in terms of growing. God is seen in terms of demand and punishment, so the disability may be considered a punishment for sins.[27]

For the person with a religion of faith, suffering can be used constructively as a means to more mature living. Guilt can be faced and confessed, and forgiveness can be accepted. Life can have meaning even though the person is permanently disabled. Often, a person with this kind of religion can move more easily through the stages of adjustment to acceptance and adaptation.[28]

Of course no one person ever fits completely into any one category, but being aware of these different concepts of religion can be useful in relating to the person and in helping him achieve a more mature and constructive view of life.

It is important for the pastor to remember that his analysis of a situation and his relationship to a person with a disability will often be done in a context other than a specific counseling situation. In fact, pastoral counseling is often lower on the list of desired services. E. Frederick Proelss has constructed a "ladder" of needs and preferences of persons with disabilities in regard to the minister. In order of preference, these services include: 1) Pastoral visitation; 2) pastoral conversation; 3) pastoral counseling; 4) group discussion; and 5) group devotions.[29] One of the most prevalent requests is to just "see" the minister, perhaps talk to him or her about religious concerns, perhaps not. The presence of the minister assures the person that he is still a valuable part of the community, and that God and the fellowship of believers have not deserted him.

In addition to relating to the individual having a disability, the minister can also play an important supportive role for the family and friends. He does so by helping them accept the reality and deal with any feelings of anger, fear, guilt, sadness, etc., that may be present. There are as many different ways for the family to respond as there are families, and their response will be as unique as will be the response of the person with the disability. The family's response depends on many factors: Whether the disability was caused by a birth defect or a later illness or accident; the extent and kind of disability; the educational and economic level of the parents; the hopes and aspirations of the parents;

the religious values and personality structures of the family.[30]

Ministry to the family is only one of the important aspects of total ministry to persons with disabilities. Another important aspect is the necessity of dealing with the community and with the problems and strengths it shows in accepting and helping people with disabilities. The minister's role in mobilizing the energies of the parish or congregation to support the persons and their families is very important. He must help the parish community develop awareness of and sensitivity toward people with many types of disabilities, and must help those people become integrated into the parish community.

Also important is the ministry he provides to the other professionals on the healing team, particularly in the institutional setting. Other members of the helping team need a chance to share concerns, support, and frustrations, if they too are to grow toward a more mature sense of values and greater affirmation of life.

The minister obviously has much to offer, both as a representative of the Church and in terms of his or her own personhood. What are some of the obstacles that the minister may have to face, and what are some of his needs as he attempts to carry out this specialized form of ministry? Some of the questions and areas of concern that the minister might have to deal with to be effective in this area of ministry are:

1. What is the minister's own emotional reaction to a person with a disability, particularly a severe, disfiguring disability? This can be a traumatic experience for any sensitive person, and can precipitate feelings of pity, revulsion, embarrassment, or threat.

2. What is the minister's own value system regarding the importance of physique and physical activities? Anyone working with persons having physical disabilities will have to come to grips with many of their own values about physical appearance, competitiveness, the work/success ethic, accomplishments in terms of physical activities.

3. What is the minister's concept of sexuality and how open is he in his ability to discuss sexual behavior and feelings? Since this is often an important problem for the disabled person and one that is difficult to discuss, the minister can offer a real service by "giving permission" to think and talk about this concern. A minister need not know all the medical terms or techniques, but can be of real service if he is aware of referral services or programs to help.

4. How honest and authentic can the minister be about his or her own negative feelings? One very real way of indicating respect for a person is by sharing true feelings. By being warm and accepting, and, at the same time, allow for expression of negative feelings (anger, disagreement, annoyance) at the appropriate times, the minister can create a positive experience for the other person. To do anything less than that is to condescend, something that will

probably be sensed by the person, and will contribute to his feelings of devaluation, inferiority, and worthlessness.

5. How comfortable does the minister feel in allowing the other person the freedom to ask questions that are really bothering him, to make his own choices, and to decide on his own values? Can the minister allow for angry feelings toward God or the Church if that is what the person is feeling, or is such a situation too threatening for the minister?

6. How knowledgeable is the minister about many different kinds of vocational, social, and psychological services that are available to help the disabled person? The minister can often do the disabled person a real service by knowing the proper agency or person to which to refer him.

7. Perhaps the most basic question is how strong is the minister's personal belief in the ascendancy of life over death and suffering? How deep is his own sense of meaning and value? How vulnerable is the minister willing to become in order to share in the struggle with depression and suffering? As was discussed earlier, the most important resource in a helping situation is the person of the helper himself and his own beliefs, values, and strengths. This is especially true as regards the minister. If he hopes to help a person through some of the really painful times in life, he must be willing to enter into that person's path, and, at the same time, maintain some degree of objectivity and offer a deep sense of hope.

Since encountering people with disabilities often brings to the foreground very deep questions about life and meaning, it is important for a person attempting to minister in this situation to have access to the support he needs as he also struggles with some of these questions.

If the minister has the strength to look at his or her own suffering and to admit his or her own personal weaknesses and disabilities, he can truly use personal wounds and suffering as a source of healing power.[31] It is at this point that the person with a disability, as well as the minister, can find the freedom to search, and through this process of searching can truly come to a point of reaffirming the value and meaning of their own lives and the worth of each individual person.

FOOTNOTES:

1. E. Frederick Proelss, "Ministering to the Physically Disabled Person," *Pastoral Psychology*, June 1965, p. 18.

2. Beatrice A. Wright, *Physical Disability: A Psychological Approach*, New York City, Harper & Bros., 1960, p. 9.

3. *Ibid.*, p. 2-3.

4. *Ibid.*, p. 9.

5. *Ibid.*, p. 87.

6. *Ibid.*, p. 92.

7. Proelss, *op. cit.*, p. 10.

8. Wright, *op. cit.*, p. 82.

9. James W. Maddock, PhD, and Deborah L. Dickman, MA (Eds.) "Sex and the Paraplegic," *Human Sexuality: A Resource Book*, University of Minnesota Medical School, Book I, Autumn 1972, no numbered pages, in section on Background and Philosophy.

10. William F. Fitzpatrick, MD, "Sexual Function in the Paraplegic Patient," *Archives of Physical Medicine and Rehabilitation*, Vol. 55, No. 5, May 1974, p. 224.

11. *Ibid.*, p. 226.

12. Proelss, *op. cit.*, p. 10.

13. Virginia Kreyer, "Feelings of Handicapped Individuals," *Pastoral Psychology*, June 1965, p. 42.

14. Wright, *op. cit.*, p. 153.

15. Kreyer, *op. cit.*, p. 42.

16. Dan H. McEver, "Pastoral Care of the Spinal Cord Injured Patient," *Pastoral Psychology*, February 1972, p. 49.

17. *Ibid.*, p. 49-50.

18. *Ibid.*, p. 50.

19. *Ibid.*, p. 52.

20. Wright, *op. cit.*, p. 112.

21. *Ibid.*, p. 114.

22. Arthur W. Combs, Donald L. Avila, and William W. Purkey, *Helping Relationships: Basic Concepts for the Helping Professions*, Boston, Allyn & Bacon, Inc., 1971, p. 3.

23. *Ibid.*, p. 15.

24. Eleanor C. Hein, *Communication in Nursing Practice*, Boston, Little, Brown, & Co., 1973, p. 170.

25. Proelss, *op. cit.*, p. 12.

26. McEver, *op. cit.*, p. 52.

27. *Ibid.*, p. 53.

28. *Ibid.*, p. 54.

29. Proelss, *op. cit.*, p. 15.

30. Eveline E. Jacobs, ACSW, "Troubled Parents: Their Feelings Toward the Handicapped," *Pastoral Psychology*, June 1965, p. 36-37.

31. Henri J.M. Nouwen, *The Wounded Healer*, Garden City, New York, Doubleday & Co., Inc., 1972, p. 84.

The Hospital Chaplain
and the Patient's Family

DAVID M. McPHEE, BA, MA, M.Div.

The scope of this article is limited to some suggestions about the pastoral theory behind support of the family of the hospital patient and some practical ways in which that support can be offered. It is not specifically concerned with the family of the terminally ill patient.

THEORY

Most people are members of a social group closely related by blood or interest. This social unit — usually, but not always, a family — is a complex entity with multiple dynamic interrelationships. The unit is often disrupted to a greater or lesser degree by the hospitalization of one of its members. A brief hospitalization may have only a slight perceptible effect; a long-term illness or a death may permanently damage it.

The process of disruption usually begins with the decision about whether or not to consult a doctor, followed by decisions concerning the most convenient time for hospitalization, if such decisions are left to the individual's discretion. Preparations for admission can be disruptive when they cause shifting of family responsibilities or roles.

It is only after hospital admission is a fact and usually after the patient is oriented to the institution, that the chaplain may become involved with the family. The chaplain is an important figure for the family since he may represent a link between normal family life and the unfamiliar, often threatening environment of the hospital. He is the only nonmedical person directly involved in patient care and has access to resources not available to other staff members. He may come into the picture in several ways.

1) Nursing personnel may ask the chaplain to see a family, because family members have become a "problem." They may be demanding, hostile, or noisy, or they may be upsetting nursing routines in some other way. Nurses may expect the chaplain to soothe and quiet disruptive people, so that the business of nursing care can go on as usual. At other times, nurses may be especially sensitive to the needs of the family and perceive the usefulness that pastoral counseling might have.

2) Physicians may ask the chaplain to help with a family. Often, at a moment of crisis, an individual doctor finds it difficult to cope with the intense emotions expressed by family members. He may ask the chaplain to come so that he can depart gracefully, either because of the pressures of time or because of his own feelings of inadequacy in dealing with this type of counseling situation.

3) The patient himself may ask the chaplain to talk with his family, usually for the purpose of improving communication. "You know how I feel about this, chaplain; can you tell my family?"

4) The family itself may seek out the chaplain for pastoral counseling, either as a result of a crisis situation precipitated by the absence of the patient from the role he usually fills, or to enhance communication. "Can you explain to Dad why we think it's best for him to be in a nursing home?"

5) The hospital chaplain may be aware of the need of his presence even though he is not asked.

FAMILY BEHAVIORAL INDICES

Usually, the chaplain will be dealing with families of patients who are in the hospital for more than a few days, or who are very sick, or who have some other "problem." People with problems invariably adjust to them, whether in a healthy or unhealthy manner. For example, one appropriate way of adjusting to a loss is by increasing activity or by temporarily using a set of avoidance mechanisms. On the other hand, permanent avoidance can be unhealthy, and, in its extreme form, can become catatonic schizophrenia. Following is a description of some of the ways people adjust to the disruption of the family occasioned by the hospitalization of one of its members.

1) An obvious way is through anger and hostility toward hospital staff members, usually expressed through accusations of neglect. Family

members trasfer their own guilt over past real or imagined neglect of the patient to the staff, at least temporarily. Since it is socially unacceptable to be angry at the patient for being absent, this anger too may be transferred to hospital staff. Guilt feelings toward the patient may be expiated by harassing the staff to provide the "best possible care" for the patient.

2) Intellectualization about the patient's illness or surgery can be healthy temporary avoidance of issues on the feeling level. It is characterized by many questions about the disease, usually asked with little or no display of emotion.

3) Refusal to discuss the patient's illness (or anybody's, for that matter) is a method of avoidance which can be healthy if it does not last for a long time and destroy communication. Families involved in this adjustment method may avoid any contact with nurses, physician, or chaplain. In extreme cases, some family members find it impossible to visit even the patient himself.

4) In attempts to avoid the fact of the patient's illness, close family members may feel guilt so acutely that they will begin to express undifferentiated feelings of worthlessness and thus become centered on themselves instead of the patient. These people may show little emotion, and other family members may feel angry because they seem unconcerned about the patient.

5) Some family members fantasize and resort to magical thinking, and some try to communicate this to the patient. Catholic chaplains in particular receive offerings for Masses, requests for many repetitions of the sacrament of the sick and for multiple baptisms of a sick child. Occasionally families will deceive a chaplain so that he will repeat sacraments already performed elsewhere. This "turning to religion" can be either healthy or unhealthy, depending on the degree of duration of the avoidance.

6) Other attempts at avoidance can be symptomatic of a preexisting disorder in the family member. Self-punitive behavior, such as all-night vigils with a patient who is not sick enough to need them, is one type. Another is the development of psychosomatic disorders similar to the disease of the patient, as a kind of attempt at expiatory avoidance.

In all of these forms of avoidance it should be remembered that many defenses are necessary and healthy, and not all should be confronted. The pastoral counselor begins by listening to feelings expressed verbally, non-verbally, or symbolically. He may help families confront their feelings and learn to short-circuit destructive ones, so that the family's supportive presence can contribute to the patient's return to health.

SOME ROUTINE PRACTICES

Every hospital chaplain has certain routine practices he feels are of value to patients' families, and other practices that he would like to implement. One such routine practice is his presence in certain areas of the hospital other than patients' rooms. Some of these areas are:

1) The emergency room. In most general hospitals, the emergency room doubles as a kind of outpatient center for minor treatment which could be performed in a physician's office. Families who bring in a member for this kind of treatment often feel that the impersonal atmosphere is more or less dehumanizing, especially when they have to wait for long periods. A concerned chaplain can help here.

Secondly, the ER is often the site of emergency cardiopulmonary resuscitation. During a cardiac emergency, family members are in crisis. The family's first concern at this time is often with knowing just what is going on. While the chaplain defers to the physician in charge of the team, the period during which the doctor is not available for communication is a critical one for the family, and even vague bits of information that team members want to pass along to the family seem of great help. If the chaplain understands the routines of the treatment, he can tell the family, in a general way, what is being done, always with tact and discretion.

In a hospital which recognizes chaplains as members of the treatment team, nurses and doctors become accustomed to the chaplain's presence and are not upset by his role in communicating with the family. Instead, they usually welcome his assistance, provided he stays out of the way of the actual treatment being given. Some medical people have commented that the treatment itself, because of its emergency nature, is dehumanizing for the patient, who is usually naked, cut, jabbed, and struck in the process. Patients may even have teeth broken or ribs cracked, injuries unavoidable because of the nature of the situation. Hopefully, the occasional presence of the chaplain serves as a quiet witness to the human dignity of the patient for skilled medical people who are too busy to think of anything other than what must be done. While this witness is more a ministry to staff members, the family of the patient may appreciate that the chaplain is present.

2) The x-ray waiting room. While emergencies do not usually occur here, the room is filled with people who are anxious about whether or not a child's arm is broken, whether a family member has a tumor, etc. In addition, some x-ray procedures are more dangerous and painful than some surgical procedures, and, while they are less understood than surgery, they may cause as much anxiety.

3) The surgery waiting room. While it is the surgeon's responsibility alone to inform the family of the outcome of an operation, the hospital chaplain can further communicate here as well. Many hospitals have a "quiet room" where patients wait on carts before surgery and receive their presurgical medications. They usually are there one hour. There is also a postanesthesia recovery room, in which patients may stay a half hour or more. Thus, a patient who has surgery lasting only 30 minutes

may be absent from his room for two hours or more, while his family waits in the surgery waiting room. Normally, the chaplain will have seen the patient and perhaps his family the evening before and thus have a kind of contact with them. His presence in the waiting room can be therapeutic for the family, particularly if he can act as a link between them and the patient in the "quiet room" or in the PAR.

Other areas in the hospital which call for the chaplain's presence include the cafeteria, where the families of long-term patients may eat regularly; the maternity waiting room, where the new father may be at any time; or even the main hospital lobby.

OTHER PRACTICAL SUGGESTIONS

1) Families should be present for anointing of the sick, and might be invited to "impose hands" on the sick person after the priest does.

2) Mass can be offered in the room of a long-term patient with the family present. I usually use a bedside stand, covered, and placed at the foot of the bed, and sometimes anoint after the Gospel.

3) If the hospital kitchen has "hospitality carts" ready for families who seem to need coffee and rolls, in addition to the concern which the cart symbolizes, they should be available at the request of a chaplain or head nurse.

4) When a patient dies, a personal letter can be sent by the hospital administration, and members of the department of pastoral care may choose to attend the wake and funeral, if any. They may also decide to telephone a surviving spouse.

SUMMARY

The chaplain has an important ministry to the families of patients. He should be aware of the kind of behavior they use to express their feelings and needs, particularly avoidance behavior. One practical way in which he can come into contact with the families — by request, or on his own initiative — is by being present and available in areas of the hospital other than patient rooms.

The Process of Dying

LEE DOUCETTE, BA

The first time I was asked if I believed a patient should be told all the facts concerning his condition, including the fact that the illness was very likely terminal, I quickly responded, "Of course." Yet with greater experience and greater exposure to the literature, I am not so certain my response was correct.

St. Augustine implied that it is only in the facing of death that man's self is born. Man can completely understand himself only by integrating the death concept into his life.

Herman Feifel[1] wrote, "Some think and say that it is cruel and traumatic to talk to dying patients about death. Actually, my findings indicate that patients want very much to talk about their feelings and thoughts about death but feel that we, the living, close off the avenues for their accomplishing this."

Feifel goes on to say, "A goodly number of terminally ill patients prefer honest and plain talk about the seriousness of their illness from their physicians. They evince a sense of being understood and helped, rather than becoming frightened or panicking, when they can talk about their feelings concerning death. . . . There is almost nothing as crushing to a dying patient as to feel that he has been abandoned or rejected. This realization not only removes a support and prevents the patient's getting relief from the guilt feelings of various kinds which he has, but does not even permit him to make use of the denial mechanisms which he may have been able to use until then. It seems that in many circumstances it is not what the patient is told, but rather how that counts. Patients can accept and integrate information that they are to die in the near future but want a gradual leading-up to this rather than a 'cold-shower' technique as one patient put it."

This view is upheld by research on this question of informing patients. Kasper[2] indicated that from 77 to 89 percent of the patients he studied said they would want to know if they were dying. Of the 60 patients studied by Feifel, 82 percent reported that they would prefer to be informed about their condition.

However, one study of physicians found that an overwhelming majority of those interviewed wanted to be informed if they had an incurable disease, but they were less willing to provide such information to others in the same situation. In research that has studied the beliefs of physicians on this point, between 69 and 90 percent of the doctors, depending on the study, did not favor telling the patient that he was dying.[3] Thus, we see that those persons in charge of patient care can develop mental blocks of their own concerning death.

Should we deliberately hold back information from the patient concerning his health status? When a patient wishes to know of the status of his condition, the physician risks certain complications by withholding information. Dr. Rothenberg[4] made the following points: "For one thing, an almost unavoidable effect of a disruptive communication is an increase in the patient's isolation and loneliness (when we hold back information on his case). Worse still, the patient may sense changes in the reactions of relatives and staff toward him and be unsure, consciously at least, of the reason for these changes."

Chapter 688 of the Minnesota state statutes require each hospital to develop a patients' bill of rights. One such document at St. Mary's Hospital, Minneapolis, states: "Every patient can reasonably expect to obtain from his physician or the resident physician of the institution complete and current information concerning his diagnosis, treatment, and prognosis in terms and language the patient can reasonably be expected to understand. In such cases that it is not medically advisable to give such information to the patient the information may be made available to the appropriate person in his behalf."

Under such conditions, the patient or his family can be reasonably certain that whatever the feelings of the physician may be they will be told the facts about the patient's condition. Yet, Feifel warns that there should be degrees of awareness. A physician should not simply burst into a patient's room and announce, "Well, I am sorry to tell you that you will die soon." There must be a gradual disclosure of the patient's true condition, and the patient should be allowed to hear what he wants to hear when he wants. As we will see when we review Glaser's awareness steps, there may well be cases where the patient prefers to be kept uninformed. The important thing to remember in this respect is that the patient should set the rules, not the doctor or nurses.

Some maintain that many patients simply cannot cope with the reality of their condition, but there is little evidence to support such a theory. The important point is that it is up to the patient to indicate whether he can or wants to face his condition realistically.

Whether we can really keep the truth from the terminally ill patient is questionable. Dr. Ross wrote that most patients know the seriousness of their case whether they are told or not. While they may not speak of their death with either doctor or relatives or friends, they know that the end is coming. Hutschnecker supports this view when he writes, "If we discount accidents and homicide, it seems to me almost certain that deep within themselves most patients know when they are going to die and most of them are ready."[5]

It can be harmful to deliberately hold back information from a patient who may want to know. Vernon and Payne wrote, "When we refuse to recognize that a person is dying, or let him know that we are aware of his dying behavior, we impose an isolation upon him. Such agreed upon silence may increase the patient's fears and despair while at the same time cutting him off from the opportunity to reduce those anxieties through sympathetic discussion or some type of therapy. Some patients suffer more from the emotional isolation and unwitting rejection than from an illness per se."[6] This view is shared by Feifel, Rothenberg, Reeves and Hinton. Hinton reported that only seven percent of the people considered in one study resented frankness when told they had cancer.[7]

On this question, it appears that the patient has the right to be informed of his condition. While the physician should provide only as much as the patient can tolerate or really wants to know, he has no right to deliberately withhold his diagnosis. Sharing such information with patients in a tactful supportive manner can be of emotional benefit to most people and can help them die with dignity.

Many patients go through a series of awareness factors. Barney Glaser and Anselm Strauss[8] have developed an awareness progression, the steps of which include:

Closed Awareness: In American hospitals, the patient frequently does not recognize his impending death even though the hospital personnel have the information. This situation can be described as a "closed awareness."

There are at least five important structural conditions which contribute to the existence and maintenance of closed awareness. First, most patients are not especially experienced at recognizing the signs of impending death. Second, American physicians ordinarily do not tell patients outright that death is probable or inevitable. Third, families also tend to guard the secret. Fourth, hospital staff members are trained to discuss with patients only the surface aspects of their illnesses, and, they are accustomed to acting collusively around patients so as not to disclose medical secrets. Fifth, the patient ordinarily has no allies who can reveal or help him discover the staff's knowledge of his impending death.

Suspicion Awareness: Often, a patient does not know, but only suspects with varying degrees of certainty, that hospital personnel believe him to be dying. The difficulty — we do not say the impossibility —of withholding information about the patient's terminality from him is recognized in American hospitals. Hospital personnel commonly subscribe to the belief that most terminal patients "really know" they are dying, whether or not they openly display that knowledge. They reason that patients must know because, given a combination of alarming symptoms, the hospitalization itself, and the many telltale cues afforded by various institutional arrangements, it is impossible for them to be unaware. Added to these factors the fact that the physician may tell the patient indirectly, by his tone of voice or his lack of optimism, and staff members reason that even if a patient does not talk about his impending death or "test" bystanders to validate his suspicions, nevertheless he must recognize that he is dying.

Mutual Pretense Awareness: When patient and staff both know that the patient is dying but pretend otherwise, a situation of mutual pretense exists. However, neither patient nor staff may be able to avoid bringing impending death into the open if radical physical deterioration occurs, the staff because it has a tough job to do and the patient for other reasons, including fright and panic. Sometimes a patient breaks his pretense when he discovers that he cannot face death alone or when a chaplain convinces him that it is better to bring things out into the open than to remain silent. Sometimes, however, a patient may find such a sympathetic listener in the chaplain that he can continue his pretense with other personnel.

For the patient, this pretense can yield a measure of dignity and considerable privacy, though it may deny him the closer relationships with staff members and family members that sometimes occur when he allows them to participate in his open acceptance of death.

Open Awareness: Whenever both staff and patient know that he is dying and acknowledge it in their actions, the context is one of open awareness. Even in this context, however, there is a holding back of certain aspects of death. Only rarely will staff members attempt to make the patient fully aware of the time and mode of death, especially if they judge the time to be sooner than the patient expects or the mode to be unpleasant. The awareness, therefore, of subsidiary features of terminality may be different than the openness about death itself.

Once a patient has indicated his awareness, he becomes responsible for his acts as a dying person. He knows now that he is not merely sick but dying, and he must face that fact. Sociologically, "facing" an impending death means that the patient will be judged, and will judge himself, according to certain standards of proper conduct. These standards pertain to the way a man handles himself during his final hours and to his behavior during the days he spends waiting to die, and they apply even to physically dazed patients. Similarly, certain standards apply to the conduct of hospital personnel, who must behave properly as humans and as professionals.

Glaser's awareness research indicates that a patient may go through one or all of these steps. His progression may be gradual or sudden. It is important to emphasize, again, that there is nothing wrong with closed awareness, as long as the patient chooses it rather than the physician. We cannot force our views on a patient merely because we think we know best.

Assuming that the patient has an open awareness of his terminal illness, what happens next. Dr. Ross reports that all of her patients reacted to the bad news in almost identical ways — ways that are typical not only in terms of fatal illness but to any great and unexpected stress: Namely, shock and disbelief. Let us examine this first reaction of the dying patient.

INITIAL SHOCK

In a paper on the psychological problems in terminal cancer management, Dr. Rothenberg[9] lists several issues which the terminal patient must resolve. This discussion of the patient's initial shock reaction includes two of his points.

Many cancer patients feel that cancer will slowly eat away at them, that they will have no control over the process, and that they will eventually loose self-control and self-mastery. According to Dr. Rothenberg this is the single most frightening aspect of his illness to a terminal cancer patient.

During the initial "panic" period, some patients try to assign blame for their plight. The patient may blame himself for not taking better care of himself, and this self-blame quickly turns into guilt. Or a patient and his family may assume a magical outlook that might be summed up in the statement, "If I don't think something or say something is so, then it isn't so." Concerning the patient's religious faith, Dr. Rothenberg writes, "Mature religious faith can be an important comfort to a dying person but a resort to a magical concept of religion is especially evident in those situations in which the patient and family reject sound medical advice because 'prayer and God will take care of things.' "[10]

Both Dr. Rothenberg and Dr. Ross discuss the denial process which is part of the initial shock phase. Dr. Ross reports that denial, or at least partial denial, is adopted by almost all patients. Such denial, at least at the outset, is good in that it provides the patient and his family with a little time to think things through. The patient may well want to be alone during this period of time, which does not mean that the patient may not want to sit and talk with someone about his impending death at some later time. However, the patient must be able to set the time for this kind of discussion.

Dr. Rothenberg pointed out, "The patient may insist that he has a curable inflammation, a precancerous lesion, or even no illness at all. He may be so convinced of this belief that he is not ill, in fact, that he rejects appropriate aid. Even patients with visible lesions or patients who have been explicitly told that they are dying of cancer adhere to such belief."[11]

Denial is one phase that probably remains with the patient off and on throughout his ordeal. Drs. Weisman and Hackett[12] state, "For the majority of dying patients, it is likely that there is neither complete acceptance nor total repudiation of the imminence of death. To deny this 'middle knowledge' of approaching death is to deny the responsiveness of the mind to both internal perceptions and external information."

During this stage it is only natural for fear to take hold. Fear of his condition and the uncertainty probably began at the time of the initial hospitalization period, and is now compounded by the fear of the loss of his own life. As Dr. Noyes[13] wrote, "Some anticipate leaving unrealized goals as they depart from this life. Others sense the emptiness of wealth and status, values that formerly gave rise to striving. Above all, dying individuals dread leaving loved ones."

Another fear that Dr. Noyes identifies is the fear of afterlife. "Death is an unknown; we are like children stumbling into the dark as we approach it. Where feelings of guilt or sinfulness are present, as they frequently are, some, according to their beliefs, grow apprehensive of possible punishment."

Dr. Ross[14] sums up this initial shock phase by saying, "What I am trying to emphasize is that the need for denial exists in every patient at times, at the very beginning of a serious illness more so than towards the end of life. Later on the need comes and goes, and the sensitive and perceptive listener will acknowledge this and allow the patient his defenses without making him aware of the contradictions. In the long run it is the persistent nurturing role of the therapist who has dealt with his or her own death complex sufficiently that helps the patient overcome the anxiety and fear of his impending death. If we are willing to take an honest look at ourselves, it can help us in our own growth and maturity. No work is better suited for this than the dealing with very sick, old, or dying patients."

Another aspect of denial is the type of encouragement the terminally ill patient receives from help-care people. Their own doubts and fears become obvious when they encourage the patient to deny the seriousness of his illness. Both Rothenberg and Glaser support this theory. Rothenberg[15] writes, "Denial of reality and especially denial of feelings can lead to severe personal and interpersonal conflicts. As will be seen in some of the clinical illustrations to follow, the house staff both deliberately and inadvertently does tend to support denial of disease and denial of angry feelings."

The family of the terminally ill patient also contributes to the phase of denial. Because of their own fears of death, family members encourage the patient to deny the seriousness of his illness, attempting to reassure themselves and the patient with such generalities as, "Everything will be all right; you have a good doctor and a good hospital."

It is difficult, however, to maintain this denial when contact with the patient confirms the opposite. Bowers[16] states, "Then it may be that a new and healthier quality comes into the relationship, and honesty with the patient makes it possible for true communication and genuine relationship to be established."

ANGER

It is only natural for a terminally ill patient to strike out over his sense of helplessness. Anger at the physician and at God is a sign of his struggle for a healthier attitude toward reality. Dr. Ross[17] has a great deal to say on this aspect of the dying process:

"In contrast to the stage of denial, this stage of anger is very difficult to cope with from the point of view of family and staff. The visiting family is received with little cheerfulness and anticipation, which makes the encounter a painful event. They then either respond with grief and tears, guilt or shame, or avoid future visits, which only increases the patient's discomfort and anger.

"The relationship between the patient and those around him or her during this period requires a tremendous amount of patience and understanding. A patient who is respected and understood, who is given attention and a little time, will soon lower his voice and reduce his angry demands. He will know that he is a valuable human being, cared for, allowed to function at the highest possible level as long as he can. He will be listened to without the need for a temper tantrum, he will be visited without ringing the bell ever so often because dropping in on him is not a necessary duty but a pleasure.

"We have to learn to listen to our patients and at times even to accept some irrational anger, knowing that the relief in expressing it will help them toward a better acceptance of the final hours. We can do this only when we have faced our own fears of death, our own destructive wishes and have become aware of our own defenses which may interfere with our patient care."

Carl Scherzer[18] offers ministers the following advice on this phase of anger, "The clergyman must not become disconcerted when a faithful one questions God's love or expresses antagonism toward the pastor which will add still another stress. The pastor's understanding and demeanor, under such conditions, communicates God's love and helps to confirm the patient's wavering faith. The pastor will be helpful by being permissive so the patient will have an opportunity to give expression to any doubts or feelings of hostility toward God. Then, with understanding and patience he may help the parishioner confirm his or her faith through counseling rather than preaching."

This is a particularly difficult time for members of the family and those who are providing care. Unless aware of this natural response, members of the family in particular may take these outbursts of anger as a personal thing. They may respond with the general attitude, "Well, if this is what he thinks of me, I'll stay home in the future." This of course would be inappropriate, and the minister should counsel the family that anger is part of the acceptance process of a terminal condition. The patient can't be abandoned, because this would only add to his depression. In a survey[19] of nurses' attitudes on this question, 83.9 percent sensed a lack of family interest, and 82.4 percent commented on the infrequency with which visitors came to see the dying patient.

GRIEF

Most people consider grieving as part of the bereavement process. However Rothenberg[20] points out that the terminally ill patient can go through a grieving process also. He writes, "The prospect of imminent death and the loss of important organs (through surgery or through disease) are undeniable causes for grieving." He goes on to say that the help-care people and the family of a terminally ill patient tend to play down this grief syndrome because, "To relatives and house staff, the patient's tears and sadness may be frightening and unacceptable."

The terminally ill patient should be allowed to freely grieve if he desires to do so. After all, the patient is losing his entire life, all his friends and relatives, all the things he likes to do and places he likes to go. The minister can assist the patient by being compassionate and understanding and by grieving along with him.

BARGAINING

Dr. Ross's book contains a short yet important chapter on the subject of bargaining. A person who is terminally ill may try to strike a bargain with God for a little additional time. The patient may have ignored his religious growth most of his life, yet at this particular time he says to himself that he will become deeply religious if God will allow him additional time. Dr. Ross[21] writes, "If we have been unable to face the sad facts in the first period and have been angry at people and God in the second phase, maybe we can succeed in entering into some sort of an agreement which may postpone the inevitable happening: If God has decided to take us from this earth and he did not respond to my angry pleas, He may be more favorable if I ask nicely."

The bargaining is really an attempt to postpone, and includes the idea of a prize offered "for good behavior." It establishes a self-imposed deadline, and it includes an implicit promise that the patient will not ask for more time if only this one postponement is granted. "Most bargains are made with God and are usually kept a secret or mentioned between the lines or in a chaplain's private office. In our individual interviews without an audience we have been impressed by the number of patients who promise "a life dedicated to God" or "a life in the service of the Church" in exchange for some additional time."[22]

DEPRESSION

"The treatment of depression in dying patients deserves greater attention. Some patients wished to talk of their problem, and experienced relief on sharing their knowledge with a person who had to do no more than accept whatever was said. Others were cheered by any companionship, for a dying patient, even amongst others, can suffer great emotional isolation and deprivation."[23] This statement refers to the depression phase through which many terminally ill patients pass.

Dr. Ross considers depression to be a normal part of the dying process. She identifies two types of depression, although the terminally ill patient is likely to be involved only in the second. The first is called reactive depression and relates to such things as possible loss of figure due to surgery, boarding out of children because of the parent's hospitalization, etc. There are specific things that can be done for the patient suffering from this type of depression. Encouragements and reassurances are useful.

When depression is used as a tool to prepare for the impending loss of all love objects in order to facilitate the state of acceptance, then encouragement and reassurance are not as meaningful. The patient should not be encouraged to look at the sunny side of things, as this would mean he should not contemplate his impending death. It would be contraindicated to tell him not to be sad, since all of us are tremendously sad when we lose a beloved person. The patient is in the process of losing everything and everybody he loves. If he is allowed to express his sorrow, he will find final acceptance much easier, and he will be grateful to those who can sit with him during this stage of depression without constantly telling him not to be sad.

This second type of depression is usually a silent one, in contrast to the first type in which the patient has much to share and requires many verbal interactions and often active interventions on the part of people in many disciplines. In the preparatory grief there is little or no need for words. It involves a feeling that can often be mutually expressed better by a touch of a hand, a stroking of the hair, or just a silent sitting together. This is the time when the patient may just ask for a prayer, when he begins to occupy himself with things ahead rather than behind.

Included in this sense of depression is what Dr. Rothenberg calls a "sense of failure": Failure on the part of the patient to seek out medical help earlier; failure on the part of the doctor to take more thorough tests to determine the problem. Everyone is looking for a scapegoat for the problem at hand. The doctor hates to admit a failure, and the patient sees failure within himself. Both doctor and patient see failure each time they see one another.

FINAL STAGE

If a patient has had sufficient time (i.e., not a sudden, unexpected death), he will probably proceed to the final stage which some have described as a phase of acceptance. It is important to point out that some terminally ill patients never get beyond the initial shock phase. They may adopt a form of denial which they carry with them to the end. But Ross, Noyes, Saunders, and others report that very few people maintain the denial phase right up to the end. Most will reach some form of acceptance. Dr. Noyes[24] reports that "as the end draws near and as emotional investment in life is withdrawn some will show, according to their faith, a growing religious concern. Faith in God may at this time develop to a high point."

Ross reports that a terminally ill patient will already have mourned the impending loss of so many meaningful people and places that he will be able to contemplate his coming end with a certain degree of quiet expectation. He will usually be tired, and in many cases, quite weak. He will also have a need to doze off to sleep during times of depression. This particular state is almost void of feelings, and it certainly shouldn't be mistaken for happiness.

About the aspect of dying, Bowers[25] writes, "The fear of death seems to exist up to a point where it is fairly close, and then gives way to a kind of peaceful understanding. This is not resignation or merely giving up. Rather it is a dim unverbalized awareness that this is a part of it all and that it does not call for terror or even real loss."

While the dying patient has found some peace and acceptance, his circle of interest diminishes. He may have said goodbye to many friends and relatives and at this point he wishes to be left alone more than in the past. It is important to remember, however, that he doesn't want to be isolated. Isolation is among the worst of human sufferings. At this point nonverbal communications may be more important than verbal.

The patient may just make a gesture of the hand to invite us to sit down for a while. He may just hold our hand while we sit with him in silence. Such moments of silence may be the most meaningful communications for people who are not uncomfortable in the presence of a dying person. Our presence may just confirm that we are going to be around until the end. Ross[26] states it well, "It may reassure him that he is not left alone when he is no longer talking and a pressure of the hand, a look, a leaning back in the pillows may say more than many noisy words."

It is during this phase that the family needs more help, understanding, and support than the patient himself. It is a particularly difficult period for those left behind. Most people find the final hours or days very taxing. Many simply cannot bring themselves to be with a dying person because of their own feelings about death.

Weisman and Hackett[27] wrote of a situation that sometimes develops. "Frequently it is the survivors who withdraw interest from the patient. The syndrome of premortem loneliness, bereavement of the dying, is partially evoked by the isolation the living force upon the dying."

This phenomenon was first expressed by Erich Lindemann who in 1944 wrote about his research with families of servicemen. Lindemann called this phase anticipatory grief. In his work with survivors Lindemann found that before the serviceman was reported killed in action, his wife or parents had separated themselves from him by going through all or many of the stages of grief including, "depression, heightened preoccupation with the departed, a review of all the forms of death which might befall him, and anticipation of the modes of readjustment which might be necessitated by it."[28]

If there has been a prolonged illness, members of the family may have already separated themselves from the terminally ill patient before the patient actually dies. This places greater emphasis on the shoulders of doctors, nurses, and ministers to work with the patient and members of the surviving family.

CONCLUSION

We have attempted to review some of the more important phases that a terminally ill patient is likely to experience before his death. All patients do not go through all these phases. Some stop at the initial shock phase, while others proceed immediately to an acceptance phase. Most, however, proceed through a number of these stages and spend varying amounts of time in each. The sensitive minister must be aware of the phases through which the patient is passing, because it is his job to guide him through these phases with understanding, empathy, and consideration. These phases are perfectly normal, and patients should be encouraged to express their feelings openly without shame or guilt.

Russell Noyes noted that in his research he found that the final time was not physically painful. This view is shared by many others. For most people, death comes peacefully. "The so-called 'death agony' really doesn't exist. Physically the dying patient may have certain muscular contortions that gives the impression of agony, yet mentally most are at peace."[29]

Noyes[30] summed up his review when he wrote, "Though death may be easy, every age has borne testimony to the profound significance of dying. It has been recognized as a potentially climactic moment in life when an individual confronts his mortality. During this moment, a man may find the opportunity to view his life in perspective and achieve previously unattained humility. He may strengthen his faith and increase his level of maturity. Dying provides a true test of an individual's beliefs, and his courage in facing death may bear witness to their strength. The person who maintains his dignity and courage while dying in effect preserves it for a lifetime and for the memory of his surviving family. In these matters the dying patient seeks the watchful eye and the guiding hand of his wise physician." Hopefully, he seeks the help of his minister also.

As for the minister's part in this journey, I believe that Henri J. M. Nouwen[31] said it well, "After so much stress on the necessity of a leader to prevent his own personal feelings and attitudes from interfering in a helping relationship, it seems necessary to reestablish the basic principle that no one can help anyone without becoming involved, without entering with his whole person into the painful situation, without taking the risk of becoming hurt, wounded or even destroyed in the process. The beginning and the end of all Christian leadership is to give your life for others. Thinking about martyrdom can be an escape unless we realize that real martyrdom means a witness that starts with the willingness to cry with those who cry, laugh with those who laugh, and to make one's own painful and joyful experiences available as sources of clarification and understanding."

FOOTNOTES:

1. Herman Feifel, "Attitudes Toward Death" in *The Meaning of Death*, Herman Feifel, ed., McGraw-Hill Book Co., Inc., New York City, 1959, p. 125.

2. August M. Kasper, "The Doctor and Death" in *The Meaning of Death*, Herman Feifel, ed., McGraw-Hill Book Co., New York City, 1959.

3. Glenn M. Vernon and William D. Payne, "Myth Conceptions About Death," *Journal of Religion and Health*, January 1973.

4. Albert Rothenberg, MD, "Psychological Problems in Terminal Cancer Management," *Cancer*, Sept.-Oct. 1961, p. 1066.

5. Arnold A. Hutschnecker, "Personality Factors in Dying Patients" in *The Meaning of Death*, Herman Feifel, ed., McGraw-Hill Book Co., New York City, 1959, p. 179.

6. Vernon and Payne, *op. cit.*, pp. 72-73.

7. J. M. Hinton, "The Physical and Mental Distress of the Dying," *Quarterly Journal of Medicine*, January 1963, p. 19.

8. Barney G. Glaser and Anselm L. Strauss, *Awareness of Dying*, Aldine Publishing Co., Chicago, 1965.

9. Rothenberg, *op. cit.*

10. *Ibid.*, p. 1064

11. *Ibid.*

12. Avery D. Weisman, MD and Thomas P. Hackett, MD, "Predilection to Death," *Psychiatric Medicine*, 1961, p. 250.

13. Russell Noyes, Jr., "The Care and Management of the Dying," *Archives of Internal Medicine*, Aug. 1971, p. 300.

14. Elisabeth Kubler-Ross, *On Death and Dying*, MacMillan, New York City, 1969.

15. Rothenberg, *op. cit.*, p. 1065.

16. Margaretta Bowers, et. al., *Counseling the Dying*, James Aronson, Inc., New York City, 1975.

17. Kubler-Ross, *op. cit.*

18. Carl J. Scherzer, *Ministering to the Dying*, Prentiss Hall, New Jersey, 1963.

19. John R. Cavanagh, "The Chaplain and the Dying Patient," *Hospital Progress*, November 1971.

20. Rothenberg, *op. cit.*, p. 1065.

21. Kubler-Ross, *op. cit.*, p. 82.

22. *Ibid.*, p. 83.

23. Hinton, *op. cit.*, p. 18.

24. Noyes, *op. cit.*, p. 301.

25. Bowers, *op. cit.*, p. 18.

26. Kubler-Ross, *op. cit.*

27. Weisman and Hackett, *op. cit.*, p. 140.

28. Erich Lindemann, MD, "Symptomatology and Management of Acute Grief," *American Journal of Psychiatry*, September 1944, pp. 147-148.

29. Cavanagh, *op. cit.*, p. 35.

30. Russell J. Noyes, Jr., "The Art of Dying," *Perspective in Biology and Medicine*, Spring 1971, p. 444.

31. Henri J. M. Nouwen, *The Wounded Healer*, Doubleday & Co., Garden City, New York, 1972.

Grief — A Common But Unique Experience

SISTER GERALDINE EAKES, OP, BS, MA

Grief is an emotion and therefore involves the feeling life of a person. Because it is experienced differently by each individual, it is hard to define or to explain to anyone else. In general, it is psychic pain which is felt deeply inside the person. Grief is a tearing kind of emotion that shuts the person off from fulfillment of hopes, dreams, and aspirations.

Grief is a normal response to a loss, because it is the other side of the coin of love. Our capacity to have deep feeling for another person is also the source of our capacity for acute pain at his loss. The fact that this capacity is proof of our highly developed nature may not make grief less painful, but it can make it more acceptable and understandable. Grief is not something to be ashamed of or something we should try to hide.

Our emotions are a vital and central part of our personality, and they become of major concern during a serious crisis. Often we have only slight awareness of how our emotions develop and of how we can meet wisely our emotional needs. Our emotional capacity for grief should not distress us: Rather, the tendency to pervert or deny our grief should be a source of concern.

Grief varies from person to person. It is a complex emotion, a composite of multiple reactions that make up the life of the grieving person. We are more emotionally dependent on others at the time of acute grief than at any other time in life, with the exception of infancy. If we can recognize this fact, we will be in a better position to accept and appreciate the help that is available. After we have been helped through the emotional crisis of grief, we can understand how important it is to be ready and willing to help others through the crises that occur in their lives.

GRIEF: WHO EXPERIENCES IT?

Grief is experienced by a person who has lost someone or something that is important to him. The intensity of the grief depends upon the significance of the loss. Significant loss is almost always experienced at the death of a loved one. In addition, some surgical procedures affect a person's body image and self-esteem to such an extent that the depression that sometimes follows radical surgery is related to unconscious grief for the lost member of the body.

Grief is inevitable. Everyone in his lifetime must from time to time confront the loss of someone or something they love. However, people who have faced up to the loss by wrestling openly and honestly with the problem have said that grief can be counted among the great deepening experiences of life.

NORMAL RESPONSES TO GRIEF SITUATIONS

A person who has just experienced a loss may be speechless, stand as if transfixed, or actually faint. These kind of responses occur especially when the bereaved person has not seen the person die, if the onset of the illness was sudden, or if an accident is involved. The initial shock is often followed by a sharp pain in the abdomen, pounding in the head, dry feeling in the mouth, palpitation of the heart, sighing, loss of appetite, or loss of awareness of surroundings. These physical manifestations may become more pronounced during the bereavement and may continue for days or even for weeks.

It is normal for the bereaved to want to talk about the deceased, to recount the circumstances preceding death, and to idealize the person. When a person is allowed to vent his thoughts and feelings in this way, he experiences a feeling of release and the beginning of acceptance of the pain of loss. The burden can be shared if the bereaved can relate the closing events and the last words with someone who will listen.

Tears are the most common expression of intense feeling or deep emotion. We should not be ashamed to show tears, nor should we deny that we have these deep feelings. A general and genuine fear is that the bereaved will become mentally ill if he gives way to grief. Precisely the opposite is true. Giving vent to feelings through tears or verbal expression is good mental health insurance.

Guilt feelings are usually expressed not so much in actions as in words, e.g., "I should have gotten Mother to the doctor sooner." The bereaved can often experience relief by verbalizing such a fault or feeling. Reaction to guilt sometimes finds expression in overspending on funeral arrangements, such as buying a very expensive casket or tombstone or by giving very generously to charitable organizations.

Hostility and resentment are a normal part of the grief process. When something precious is taken from us, we react initially by being very critical of everyone related to the loss. We become critical in an attempt to understand why this thing happened and who is to blame. Such hostility and resentment must be faced if they are to be overcome.

Another normal response to grief is to entertain simultaneous negative and positive feelings about the person both before and after death. These intense emotions are aroused by the same individual simultaneously. For example, the bereaved may be bitterly accusatory: "Why did you have to die and leave me?" and yet tenderly ask, "How can I ever go on to face life without you?" Expression of such contradictory feelings can be a step toward normalcy.

Grief may have an anticipatory character. Relatives may anticipate the death of a person so much that in their minds they have already buried the person before he actually dies. Thus, they have already gone through the whole grief process before the death. Observers may report a tearless grief reaction, and the survivors themselves are puzzled by their apparent lack of grief.

THE MEANING OF A FUNERAL

The funeral is a means of expressing sorrow in a direct manner, and it has a therapeutic significance. It provides a necessary outlet for strong emotion and also an opportunity for sharing the loss in a manner that is socially acceptable. Most people have to talk out the loss before they feel free. The old custom of the family wake served this function by drawing relatives closer as they shared their loss in each other's presence through long hours of talking.

Funerals provide the community with an opportunity to express its concern. The Church, through its members, helps by sharing the burden. Grief sufferers need both sympathy and empathic care, the warmth and companionship of unhurried relationship. They need friends who do not run from cirses, friends who are aware that they are experiencing loneliness and isolation, physical and spiritual fatigue.

THE GRIEF PROCESS

Grief is a process and it takes an individual time to work through the several stages of sorrow. The first stage involves the painful task of facing the full reality of what has happened. There is usually no easy way to face the death of one who was deeply loved. The pain and the loss must simply be accepted, but the expression of feeling is of the utmost importance. One must be able to say that it hurts and be able to feel the hurt keenly to the very depth of his being. Such expression of feeling has a healing effect. However, accepting the reality of death does not usually come immediately. It takes time, frequently from three to six months.

The second stage of the grief process involves breaking some of the bonds that tie us to the person who has died. Sometimes this is called reinvesting emotional capital, because it involves translating the relationship from presence to memory. Again, this is facilitated by expressing authentic feelings in an effort to understand and deal with them. Many people find it difficult to find someone willing to share their grief. In such cases, the pastor has an opportunity to fill the role of listener.

The third stage entails finding new interests, new satisfactions, and new creative activities. In this respect, the bereaved should make new acquaintances and should establish new relationships. Memories may be treasured, but one cannot live on memories alone and remain healthy.

Sorrow is so much a part of life that we do not really begin to live until we have learned the art of dealing with sorrow creatively. Some persons allow sorrow to make them bitter and disillusioned. They are destroyed by sorrow and lose faith in everything. Others gain a new sensitivity and a deep, rich faith through the wise handling of grief. They develop understanding and more genuine sympathy for others.

RELIGIOUS RESOURCES IN THE GRIEF PROCESS

Jesus once said: "Blessed are they that mourn for they shall be comforted." Religion can provide such comfort by helping the grief sufferer recognize the need for perspective, for spiritual values, and for inner strength. Religious institutions point to values that are timeless. They emphasize the rest of life as the setting within which tragic events take their appropriate place. They seek to restore clear vision.

One of the important functions of religion is to help the grief sufferer refocus his thinking on the values that death cannot destroy. Religious beliefs include a promise of a continued life of the spirit. Religious teaching helps link the grief sufferer with things rooted in the past, things that remain unchanged in the midst of change. It ties a person to eternal things when he most needs this bond.

In worship the grief sufferer can be alone with his deepest sorrow and at the same time be surrounded and supported by others who share a common heritage and a similar spiritual concern. The quiet serenity of a place of worship has healing power. The grief sufferer's tumult is stilled and turbulent emotions are calmed by the reassurance of eternal things. Religion helps a person to look up and out, to arrive at a new perspective of life in working through the grief process.

DESTRUCTIVE WAYS OF HANDLING GRIEF

Overactivity is a form of denial of grief. Busyness can be an attempt to evade a realization of the loss. The grief sufferer attempts to blot out the image of the deceased, sometimes by discarding or burning pictures, but such dramatic gestures only seem to accentuate the loss.

Sometimes the grief sufferer will evidence physical symptoms. The common physical symptoms of unresolved grief are similar to the symptoms of arthritis and rheumatism and of colitis and other psychosomatic disorders.

Another manifestation of distorted grief is the withdrawal from social relationships. The grief sufferer will avoid social contacts, especially any activity in which the deceased had participated or which the deceased and survivor shared together. The survivor may also attempt to take up the occupation of the deceased, often failing miserably.

Potentially dangerous grief reactions usually show up in extremes. Sometimes a person feels he is no longer of value as a person and he makes veiled threats of self destruction. A person may act in a manner inconsistent with his usual behavior. For example, he may demonstrate excessive hostility or engage in excessive drinking. Or he may exhibit other antisocial behavior, withdraw completely, and no longer interact with others. A person may even flee reality by a sudden decision to fly to some remote place. When grief situations go beyond the pastor's ability and knowledge to deal effectively with them, he should refer the grief sufferer to a psychiatrist or member of the mental health team.

THE PASTOR'S ROLE

The pastor has a unique relationship to the grief sufferer. No one escapes coming to grips with the loss of loved ones through death or other forms of crises such as rejection or separation. Faced with such loss, many people have a natural inclination to turn to the pastor during this time of crisis. His manner of handling grief situations can prove decisive in the recovery of equilibrium. The presence of the pastor can symbolize a profound hope that is difficult to verbalize, the fact that God does not forsake His children in the most critical periods of their existence. The image of the pastor is one that exemplifies the spirit of Him who came to comfort and to heal broken relationships.

However, before a pastor can help others, he must know himself operationally. This includes honestly facing up to himself, knowing his strengths, weaknesses, resources, limitations, hostilities, basic anxieties, etc. It involves self-study, and self-understanding. Self-knowledge is necessary for both professional and psychological survival.

In his role as counselor, the pastor represents a measure of emotional security in a framework of unstable things. The pastor can help the grieving person deal with his problems wisely: He can help him face the reality of his situation, think through the deeper meanings of his new responsibilities, and establish new relationships. Unresolved grief complicates life; the part the pastor plays determines to a great extent how soon and how well the grief sufferer works through the grief process.

The pastor should accept the feelings of the mourner and encourage him to express his feelings of whatever kind. Tears are soothing in and of themselves. Trying to cheer up a person who has suffered a significant loss is a harmful approach. The reality and the pain of the loss must be faced and accepted. False consolations are also to be avoided. There is a common element in death, but the significant fact is the uniqueness in the common.

Prayer, scripture, and the sacraments are some of the pastor's religious resources for ministering to the grief sufferer. In the use of prayer and the selection of scripture, the guiding principle is to keep the grief sufferer close to reality without withdrawing from the pain. Prayer and scripture passages should face realistically "the valley of the shadow of death" and, at the same time, emphasize God's nearness. In the acute phase of bereavement, prayer should be brief. In its wording, it should gather up the family's feelings and recognize the course of the normal grief process. After expressing the reality of the loss and the pain of separation, the prayer should acknowledge the need for divine strength and courage during the time of bereavement.

It is not without reason that the community entrusts the care of the grief sufferer to religious leaders. The pastor's experience with life and death, his understanding of people, and his faith make him competent to help a grief sufferer emerge from the depths of his grief.

Grief may be one of the most deeply disturbing emotional states a person endures. To relieve the pain, to ease the misery of the grief sufferer is a responsibility and a privilege not to be taken lightly. To grow in competence in meeting the needs of the sorrowful is certainly one of the major tasks of the minister.

Ministry to the Elderly During Relocation

CAROLYN A. KOCHEL, RN, MS
THE REV. SAMUEL S. KOCHEL, BA, M.Div.

For many elderly persons, discharge from the hospital does not mean returning to their own homes and familiar surroundings. Rather, it means separating themselves from all that is familiar and entering an institution for the long term care of the elderly. Some of the elderly have anticipated this change as a result of gradually deteriorating health. However, others may have been healthy until a sudden illness required hospitalization, and thus may not have anticipated needing long term care in an institution. Whatever the individual's circumstances, accepting the reality of entering an institution can represent a major crisis. The hospital chaplain is an essential member of the patient care team and can make a unique contribution toward meeting the needs of the elderly during this period of transition.

VIEWS OF AGING

The way in which a person perceives and responds to this relocation is closely related to his own experiences with aging: How he feels about himself, how others respond to him, and the degree to which he feels he can be a contributing member of society.

American society, with its emphasis on change and new ideas, does not give high prestige to the elderly who generally no longer play an important role in a rapidly changing society. However, most Americans feel the elderly should be honored and respected. This ambiguity is not peculiar to our culture. Even in classical literature, we find two opposing views of aging. The Greeks placed high value on the qualities of youth, and saw no value in life after youth and vigor faded. This is contrasted with the Middle Eastern view of old age as the pinnacle of life, characterized by wisdom and virtue.

The conflict between the realities of a technological age and a desire to value the elderly is reflected in the varying ways the elderly view the process of aging and their own experience of it. To many people being old means being crippled, sick, hard of hearing, forgetful, and dependent. For others it means a time to reflect on the past and impart wisdom to others. For still others getting old may mean nothing more than white hair and glasses.[1]

Studies have shown that many people over 65 don't consider themselves old until this awareness is forced on them either by their failing health or by the way others treat them.[2] Hospitalization followed by discharge to a nursing home inescapably confronts these people with the awareness of being old.

As difficult as it is to accept decreasing physical powers and increasing infirmity, it is even more devastating to face the implication of uselessness and worthlessness. Many of the elderly feel as though they are at the mercy of others for the opportunity to maintain a role in human society. For the person who already feels useless, entering a nursing home is the final admission that there is nothing left he can do. Thus it is crucial to realize that the adjustment many persons have to make goes well beyond accepting the fact of institutional living. For many, it means facing the fact that they are old, and how they respond is directly related to what being old means to them.

For some persons the experience of aging can be characterized by three phases.[3] The initial stage involves adjusting to the role of an ager. For many, this initial stage occurs during the transition from full-time employment to retirement. Their usual life pattern and source of satisfactions are disrupted, and they must find other ways to meet their need for satisfying experiences. This transition is followed by a time when they find many opportunities for satisfaction as a healthy active elderly person. Eventually, however, health fails, and these satisfying activities have to be given up. The elderly person may then enter a third phase, a time when he feels ready to die.

For many of the elderly, their admission to the hospital heralds the beginning of this third phase, and they accept it with a sense of timeliness since they feel ready to die. However, the wonders of modern science enable some of them to get "better," and instead of dying they continue to live on. For some, this means an opportunity to resume their previous life styles. For others, however, this living on means living in a nursing home rather than returning to what they consider to be a satisfactory life style. Thus, they may see their extended life as a burden rather than an opportunity. One elderly patient stated, "I was almost gone and they brought me back. What is there left for me? I wish they had let me die. I was ready."

Other elderly persons never change their view of themselves as worthwhile contributing persons. For them, aging merely changes the nature of some of their contributions; it does not rob them of the possibility of being useful. These kind of elderly persons regard the move to a nursing home as a change of residence rather than an end to meaningful existence.

These different views of aging are given not as diagnostic categories, but as examples of the broad range of attitudes and responses evidenced by the elderly. What is important for all who work with the elderly during their transition to a nursing home is to discover what aging means to each individual in order to decide how best to meet that person's needs as he faces leaving the hospital to enter a nursing home.

NEEDS DURING RELOCATION

The specific needs that must be met throughout relocation vary from individual to individual and depend on each person's background and past experiences. There are, however, certain fundamental needs that are common to the elderly in all cultures:

1. To be recognized as a unique person with inherent worth.
2. To know that there are others who care about his welfare.
3. To exercise independence and control over his own life.
4. To feel that there is some purpose and usefulness in his existence.[4]

The intensity of these needs and the emphasis on some rather than others varies from person to person, and even from time to time for the same person.

Someone asked an elderly lady to describe the needs of the elderly. She replied, "We need what every human being needs — enough money to meet our expenses, to be able to pay the doctor when we are sick, a place to live, something to do, someone to do for, and someone to care."[5]

The elderly perceive the major threats to meeting these needs as those involving desertion, disability, suffering, and death.[6] A common theme is that of loss: The death of a spouse, loss of employment and decreased income, decreased vigor, and working out satisfactory living arrangements. All of these problems require the elderly to make adjustments in their attitudes and ways of life.

The decision to enter a nursing home involves many of these threats. It means leaving familiar surroundings for a foreign environment where the person encounters new relationships, expectations, and patterns of living. He faces a dual adjustment that would be stressful for even the most adaptable person. He must adjust to being separated from his home, family, and community, and, at the same time, adjust to group living.

Many elderly persons consider an institution an unavoidable last resort, not a welcome place of refuge. Entering a nursing home may make a person feel that he has failed to maintain himself with some degree of independence in the community. He may feel that the members of his family are abandoning him to the mercy of strangers, no longer wanting to care for him now that his health has deteriorated. Even though he may clearly recognize the fact that he needs to be cared for and although he may sincerely not want to be a burden on his children, he still has trouble ridding himself of the feeling that he is being rejected.

One of the greatest threats is the fact that frequently the decision to move a patient to a nursing home is made without consulting the patient himself. It is not uncommon on the day before discharge for someone to announce to the patient that he will be going to a nursing home and that everything has been arranged. Imagine the shock and disbelief the patient experiences. Even worse, this approach tells the patient loudly and clearly that he is no longer responsible for his own life — others have assumed control. He has been judged incapable of choosing what is best for himself, and others have taken over the task. One elderly man described his feelings when this happened to him: "They came in and told me I wouldn't go home and had to go to a nursing home. They didn't give me a chance, they just told me. Why couldn't they give me the facts and let *me* decide? I maybe would have made the same decision, but I still have the *right* to decide for myself."

ADJUSTMENTS FACING THE INDIVIDUAL

Entering the hospital requires the elderly person to make a great many adjustments, some of which are similar to those that must be made in entering a nursing home. However, there is a difference in impact in entering these two institutions. The hospital is viewed as a temporary arrangement, and this makes some of the changes seem less overwhelming. "After all, I'll only be here a while." For most people, however, the move to a nursing home involves a sense of finality: It's the last stop. It's not a question of tolerating a few temporary differences, but rather a question of adapting to a permanent or long-term living arrangement.

Some of the activities which demand adjustments when entering an institution are: Sharing a room, functioning as part of a community, accepting medical management, accepting changes in staff assignments, expressing positive and negative feelings, accepting the present living arrangements, participating in mass activities, accepting the judgment of staff members, accepting mass prepared food, living by routine, planning for the future, accepting group decisions, facing the end of life, accepting the limits of the home, accepting one's self, maintaining positive relations with family and friends, and accepting other residents. Some of these adjustments will be more stressful than others, but the overall impact is obvious.[7] The person must find a way to accommodate himself to a setting that has its own norms, values, and social structure without losing his sense of individuality and uniqueness.[8]

EXPERIENCES DURING TIME OF TRANSITION

One way of viewing the experience of transition from community to institutional living or from a hospital to an institution, is in terms of the personal meaning it has for the individual. These personal meanings may reflect feelings of desertion or fear of death, but are unrelated to the actual characteristics of the particular institution he is entering.

A second way of describing the impact of the transition is in terms of the necessary adaptation which is demanded by an environment that requires new behavior patterns. This adaptation may be very stressful since it involves abandoning familiar ways of behaving and of learning new ways to obtain gratification.

In the period of time between knowing that he will be entering a nursing home and the time the move actually occurs, the elderly person may be actively engaged in trying to work through the symbolic meaning the anticipated move will have on his own self-concept. For women, this meaning seems to center around the theme of rejection, and they are therefore concerned with constructing a new self-image within the new environment. For men, the threat is chiefly to their sense of competence and potency. They are therefore concerned with establishing an identity and image of competence within the demands of the new environment.

During this time of waiting to enter the nursing home, these persons exhibit very high anxiety levels, experience a sense of helplessness and powerlessness, appear to withdraw from relationships, have a general mood of depression, and have very little ability to look into the future.[9]

Admission to the nursing home usually involves a period of impact or shock, during which the reality of his situation temporarily immobilizes the elderly person. This period carries hazards of its own.

Research has demonstrated that the first year following an aged person's relocation, particularly the first three months, is extremely hazardous to survival. Evidence also indicates that this hazard to survival cannot be solely attributed to a weakened physical state. In cases where elderly persons have been able to adequately adapt to their previous setting, the crucial factor in their ability to survive the relocation seems to be their affective, not their physical, state. Persons who are depressed suffer extremely high risk during relocation. These people see no possibility for a satisfying future, or they see no future at all. For many, depression about the future is compounded by a lack of what they consider to have been a satisfying past. In such cases, the absence of pleasant memories or future hopes to bridge the current painful situation makes the stress of relocation total and unrelieved.[10]

One study found that the psychological factors which had a positive influence on survival were having flexible patterns of adaptation and the capacity to express anger and apprehension. Patients who reacted to the change with regression, depression, or denial had a significantly higher mortality rate.[11]

Other factors that are directly related to adjustment to institutional living are preadmission preparation of the person as to what to expect in the nursing home, and, equally important, the physical aspects and psychosocial atmosphere of the institution the person is entering.[12]

MINISTRY DURING RELOCATION

Ministering to the elderly person as he experiences the crisis of relocation to a nursing home is both an opportunity and a challenge to the hospital chaplain. The recommendations made in this section for planning pastoral care of the elderly during relocation are meant to be used with elderly persons who are coherent and alert and are based on the following beliefs about them:
1. Each aged person has the right to make his own decisions concerning what will best meet his own needs.
2. Each person's perception of relocation and his concerns regarding it are unique to him.
3. An elderly person is capable of understanding and adapting to the stresses that occur in his life.
4. The role of the chaplain is to support and assist the aged person as he decides where he will go and as he adjusts to his new environment.

MINISTRY WHILE DECISION IS MADE

It is essential not to lose sight of the fact that an aged person is a mature responsible adult. Of course, there are exceptions to this rule, situations in which senility or other mental dysfunctions prevent the person from being able to make responsible decisions. But for the majority of the elderly, their deteriorating health and decreased ability to care for some of their physiological needs does not alter the fact that they are capable of deciding how their needs can best be met.

Often members of the family and/or health team, fearing that the elderly person will make the "wrong" decision, decide for him where he will go. Frequently, the aged person learns of their decision only after all arrangements are made and the move is about to occur. This approach magnifies the aged person's feelings of helplessness and hopelessness and tells him clearly that he is no longer being considered a mature, responsible adult.

Various studies have shown that elderly persons who actively participate in the decision to enter the nursing home are far more successful in adapting to the new environment and have a more positive concept of self and attitude towards life than those who do not participate in the decision. In conversations with nursing home residents, this difference is striking. Persons who are there because they personally decided that it was best for them view themselves as competent and able to meet their needs within the nursing home setting. Residents who did not participate in the decision to enter describe themselves and their lives as helpless and hopeless, and they convey an air of depressed resignation.[13] This data indicates that participation in this decision has implications for survival, as well as for the person's outlook on life. As was cited earlier, elderly persons who are very depressed are far more likely to die during the crucial first three months after entering the home.

Two factors seem to be operative in cases where the decision is made without consulting the patient himself. First, those making the decision are concerned with making sure that the elderly person receives the care he needs. Secondly, family members, for a variety of reasons, may not want to provide the care. Notwithstanding these concerns, responsibility for deciding where another person should go violates that person's fundamental human rights. Although it is natural to care about what happens to another person, no one else can decide what is best for that person.

The elderly patient who will require long term care will need accurate information before he decides how he wants to have this care provided. First, he needs information related to his physical state: What kind of care will he require, for how long, and the alternative ways of obtaining it. He also needs to know the financial implications of the various alternatives. It is important that his family be open about their own feelings, concerns, and resources. Based on this information, the patient can determine his priorities and decide how he wants to meet his needs.

If the patient's decision requires the involvement of his family or community resources, the people who will be involved must decide whether or not they will participate. For example, if the patient decides to go home and hire a nurse to care for him and if he has the financial resources to do so, he can proceed with his plan. If, however, the patient wants his family to pay for the care, they must decide whether they are willing to do this.

The chaplain can be involved during this decision-making process in a variety of ways. Family members may need a great deal of support in deciding to allow the elderly person to make a decision for himself. Communication between the patient and his family is essential. The family needs to share their concerns, and also to be honest about the type and amount of support they are willing and able to provide the patient when he leaves the hospital. It is essential for the patient to have this information as he makes his decision.

The family may feel guilty about the amount of support they are willing to provide, and may need a lot of encouragement from the chaplain to honestly assess their own needs and strengths. Both the elderly patient and his family must accept the fact that, although they have sincere concern for each other's welfare, they are responsible for their own decisions. For example, if a daughter believes that bringing her mother home with her would exhaust her own physical and emotional reserves and thus adversely affect her marriage and her children, she has the right to make that decision. Unless she can be open and honest with her mother, the relationship between them will be seriously affected at a time when her mother needs emotional support very much.

If family members do not deal honestly with their guilt feelings, they may cope with the situation in ways which will have negative consequences for the patient. Family members may cope by attempting to avoid the situation altogether, and, thus, they stop coming to see the patient. Or they may avoid dealing openly with the patient by arbitrarily arranging for him to go to a nursing home rather than honestly discussing the situation with him. The chaplain must confront the family with the consequences of such behavior. It may be necessary for him to arrange an opportunity for the patient and family members to sit down together and discuss their feelings, with the chaplain present to provide support and to clarify areas of confusion or disagreement.

The patient also needs support during this time. He may feel rejected, abandoned, afraid, or a whole variety of emotions, and he may need the chaplain's assistance in dealing with his feelings. These feelings are a natural response to what is happening, and are part of the necessary grieving for the past that must be done before the elderly person can begin to look toward the future again. However, the patient must begin to resolve these feelings if he is going to be able to adapt positively to his new environment.

CONCERNS AND ADJUSTMENTS RELATED TO ACTUAL TRANSITION

If the decision-making process results in the conclusion that the nursing home is the best alternative, a new phase of the relocation process begins. As the elderly person begins to examine what this change will mean in his life, he needs opportunities to express and accept his feeling about moving to a nursing home.

The elderly person grieves over all that he feels he will lose in entering a nursing home. Even though he knows the move is going to happen and has accepted it as the best way to meet his needs, he still grieves as he faces the change. This is a normal response, and occurs in varying degrees and for varying periods of time for different individuals.

Many elderly persons need help in expressing their feelings and moving through the grief process, so that they can begin to see the options that will be open to them in this new setting and effectively use their new environment to meet their own needs. Many of the elderly find the chaplain or pastor to be the most helpful resource person during this time. In other instances, the family may be best able to offer support to the elderly person. In such cases, the chaplain's role would be to offer support to the family during this time. The important thing is for the elderly person to have the support of persons significant to him during this period of transition and grieving.

It is very important for the chaplain and others working with the patient to be skilled in ascertaining the patient's own perception of his condition. Often, the relationship established between the chaplain and the elderly patient during his hospitalization has been strengthened by the chaplain's supportive role during the decision-making process. Now it is essential for the chaplain to spend time sitting with and listening to the patient. Open-ended questions, clarification, and active listening are essential communication skills at this time.

Some elderly persons consider it important to be able to bring along a few personal belongings. Nothing can alter the pain of leaving one's own home and the possessions of a lifetime, but a favorite picture or chair or lamp may help some people feel a little more at home. Some persons may consider a private room crucial to maintain a sense of autonomy. Others, however, may welcome the companionship of a congenial roommate.

Once a clear picture of the patient's fears and hopes is obtained, a specific plan can be developed to meet the patient's needs during and after the actual move. This plan should involve the patient and the health care team at every step. It's important to check with the patient to make certain that the needs identified by the health care team are really the ones that are important to the patient. Before any plans are implemented, they should be discussed with the patient to ascertain whether they are acceptable to him and will effectively meet his needs.

One of the primary fears of many elderly facing relocation is the fear of the unknown.[14] Unless the patient has prior knowledge of the nursing home he will be entering, his inability to visualize his future surroundings causes unnecessary anxiety. A visit to the home, reports from relatives, or even pictures would help the patient visualize his future surroundings.

The patient's curiosity about the people he will be living with and those who will be caring for him may often be more important to him than the physical surroundings. It is not uncommon for an elderly person to have a lengthy hospitalization before he is discharged to the nursing home. During this time, he may establish close relationships with many hospital staff members. Leaving these people who have been so supportive may compound the patient's feelings of loss. One elderly man said with tears in his eyes, "How will I get along without all of you to be with me? I'm going to miss you so much."

During the waiting period, it would be very helpful if the patient could meet and get to know some of the staff and, if possible, some residents of the nursing home. Then, when the move is made, he would already have developed some relationships, and these new friends would provide support during the getting acquainted process.

The chaplain should explore the spiritual care resources available in the nursing home. Some homes have resident chaplains, while others are served by local clergy. Whichever the case, the chaplain should establish contact with the appropriate person and share whatever information about the patient he feels is relevant with whoever will be ministering to the patient. It would be helpful if the nursing home chaplain or pastor could meet the patient while he is still hospitalized, so that they could begin to establish a relationship before the move occurs. In this way, the patient would know he has someone he can call on to minister to his spiritual needs after he leaves the familiar surroundings of the hospital.

Just as the nursing home chaplain enters the picture while the patient is still in the hospital, so also the hospital chaplain may want to maintain contact with the patient for a few weeks after he moves to the nursing home. However, the crucial concern is for the nursing home chaplain to establish a close relationship with the patient, since he will be the patient's primary resource in the future.

Just as successful adjustment to living in a nursing home appears to be related to having participated in the decision to go there, feelings of independence and control over one's life appear to be vitally important in determining whether the elderly person sees himself as a person of worth or as helpless and hopeless.

Most elderly persons feel overwhelmed by the prospect of entering the nursing home, because they will be removed from all their previous ways of meeting their own needs. However, they still have some options and choices, and the task is to help them identify these choices and encourage them to exercise their options. Two people in identical situations may see themselves functioning within these limitations very differently.

In asking several nursing home residents about their ability to meet their own needs, two men were asked if they could get an aspirin for themselves if they needed one. The first man replied "No. I'd have to ask someone to get it for me." The second man replied "Yes, all I have to do is ask. . . ." The one man viewed himself as helpless because he couldn't actually get the aspirin. The second man viewed himself as being in control, because he can ask for what he needs and thus get it. This example illustrates the kind of viewpoint that elderly residents of nursing homes need to develop. Although they are no longer able to personally do certain things for themselves, they still have some control over getting what they need.

The chaplain can facilitate the development of this positive point of view in a variety of ways. He can point out situations in which the patient may not be aware of having choices. The elderly person needs to recognize choices he does have. As he recognizes these, he will become more aware of additional opportunities to exercise control over his situation.

A positive point of view can also be fostered by having a resident with a positive self-concept spend time with the patient and share some of his own experiences with him. There are times when the patient will listen to someone who is in a similar situation to the one he is facing more readily than he will listen to someone who does not share his plight.

A third possibility is to form groups of patients who will be discharged to a nursing home, to share their feelings of grief and despair and to support each other in their attempts to build or maintain a positive self-concept as they enter this new environment.

No one approach can meet the needs of each elderly person entering a nursing home. Just as each person is a unique individual, his needs are also unique. The goal of all who work with the elderly during relocation should go beyond merely ensuring survival. In this life experience, as in all others, there is the potential for personal growth and reintegration on a higher level. Entering a nursing home can be the end of the road or it can be an opportunity to build on old strengths and develop new ones in response to the challenge of a new environment. This, then, is the challenge: To ascertain from the person's attitudes if growth is possible or has occurred, and to marshal environmental and personal support for his efforts.

Perhaps one way to evaluate growth is in terms of morale. If the elderly person who enters a nursing home is able to reorganize his life in such a way that he perceives it to be meaningful and satisfying, he has emerged from the relocation crisis with the ability to cope positively with his changed existence.

FOOTNOTES:

1. Susan Pulkkinen, "A Focus on Feelings," *Nursing Outlook*, Dec. 1969, p. 71.

2. Joseph Drake, *The Aged in American Society*, Ronald Press, New York City, 1958, p. 18.

3. Dorothea Jaeger and Leo Simmons, *The Aged Ill*, Appleton-Century-Crofts, New York City, 1970, p. 7-10.

4. Carolyn Kochel, "An Exploratory Study of How Nursing Home Residents Perceive Certain Basic Needs Can Be Met," Master's Thesis, University of Minnesota, 1973, p. 1.

5. Minna Field, *Aging with Honor and Dignity*, Charles H. Thomas, Springfield, Ill., 1968, p. 11.

6. Sidney Levin, "Depression in the Aged," in *New Thoughts on Old Age*, ed. Robert Kastenbaum, Springer, New York City, 1964, p. 182.

7. Herbert Shore, "Evaluation of Self Surveying in the Modern Institution," in *Social Welfare of the Aging*, Jerome Kaplan and Gordon Aldridge, eds., Columbia University Press, New York City, 1962, p. 19.

8. Theodore Rosen, "The Resident's Adjustment to the Home," in *Geriatric Institutional Management*, eds. Morton Leeds and Herbert Shore, Putnam's Sons, New York City, 1964, p. 120.

9. Morton Lieberman, "Factors in Environmental Change," *Patterns of Living and Housing of Middle Aged and Older People*, Public Health Service Publication, No. 1496, 1965, p. 122.

10. *Ibid.*, p. 120.

11. C. Knight Aldrich and Ethel Menakoff, "Relocation of the Aged and Disabled: A Mortality Study," *Journal of the American Geriatric Society*, March 1963, p. 193.

12. Mary Fussell, "Newly Admitted Geriatric Patients Adjustment to Institutional Living," *ANA Clinical Sessions*, 1969, p. 140.

13. Alice Swan, "An Exploratory Study of How Nursing Home Residents Perceive Nursing Home Placement," Master's Thesis, University of Minnesota, 1973.

14. Louis Novick, "Easing the Stress of Moving Day," *Hospitals*, Aug. 1967, p. 69.

Christian Presence

THE REV. REX KNOWLES, PhD

In the final analysis, pastoral care is the responsibility of every person in the Church. Although there is definitely a need for full-time "professionals" who have special skills in this field, these professionals can never replace the caring of individuals from all walks of life.

Members of the health care professions must recognize how essential it is for each and every one of them to be a "general practitioner" in pastoral care. Many of us have resigned our pastoral tasks, but the time has come to re-enter pastoral work and to recognize again how important this function is. Although Glasser, Freud, Perls, Adler, Moreno, Rogers, and Skinner have all made marvelous contributions, what they have to offer can never replace pastoral care of the importance of Christian presence.

For illustrative purposes, let us consider the problem of a disturbed child. A disturbed child has suffered impaired growth, because somewhere in his development he has begun to doubt himself. He hasn't been able to grow with his experiences. His basic problem is a loss of self, and his basic suffering comes from the shattering of self-reliance. Consequently, he begins to develop defenses, and these defenses eventually become a way of life.

What kind of person can help this child? For one thing, the person who can help him must be a whole person himself. He must *be there*, and not be merely a conglomeration of theories and techniques. Rather, he must demonstrate real Christian presence. By this, I don't mean anything doctrinal. Rather, this presence refers to a sharing of self which can lead to a growth experience.

A human organism becomes a person through interpersonal relationships; through "significant others," we grow. If the "others" are warm, trusting, patient, noncontingent and rewarding — rewarding for being, not just doing — we grow into selfhood. The child who grows up in a world which is trustworthy can be warm and giving himself. If, however, his world seems untrustworthy, because people do not give and he doesn't experience warmth and love, the child learns to survive as best he can by developing defenses. What the person with Christian presence can bring to him is warmth and trust and love. Even though there is no assurance that this greater warmth, trust, patience, and love will fill the void or obliterate the defenses, there is no other way.

In attempting to develop Christian presence, it is important that we remember who we are. I am a child of God. I am sustained in my very being by divine power and love. I'm not justified by success or popularity. I'm not called to be successful; I'm called to be obedient. I am to love as I am loved. Yet, my joy is to remind that other person: "You are a child of God." I can do this in different ways, through words and doctrines, but I can also do this by the way I relate to that person, the way I love that person, the way I am — as a Christian — to him.

The essential thing in developing Christian presence is to truly live and trust and love, and to recognize and identify the nobility of others. For instance, when we walk into a hospital room to see a person, our very presence lets them know they are not alone. Certainly, this experience can be enhanced by what we say and how we say it, but basically it is our presence that gives comfort. What our presence says to the patient is: "You are a child of God and you are important."

Although this reaching out to others can, at times, be a joyful experience, at other times it can be just plain hard work. People are often engaged in a struggle for identity and a feeling of self-worth, and they may give vent to that struggle in very down-to-earth ways. Despite the difficulties we may encounter in reaching out to these people, we are obliged to help to convince them — by word and action, by our presence — that they are truly God's children and our brothers and sisters. They are a part of the Church and they evidence, in their very selves, the power of God. It is this truth that we must help them see.

We don't have to be perfect before we can be pastors. We all have our own weaknesses to contend with, but our own sinfulness cannot stand in the way of our pastoral work. If we wait until we're perfect, we'll never be pastors. Rather, Christ is calling us right now to bestow our gift of Christian presence and to exercise our greatest pastoral skill — listening.

It may take some effort to master the skill of listening, but this effort is well worth the dividends it earns. Being able to talk to a responsive listener often helps the patient see his own travail and work through to his own solutions. Of course, this cannot happen if we — not the patient — are doing all the talking. Rather, we must learn to listen responsively, offering encouragement when necessary and reacting with our feelings as much as with our words. Listening responsively represents an effort at entering the other person's inner world. We respond from where he is rather than from where we are. This requires discipline to listen without interfering, without offering advice, without comment of any kind, at times. But this kind of discipline pays off.

In our attempts to evidence Christian presence through responsive listening, we must be aware of the kinds of things that retard communication and the building of healthy relationships. Two major problems that may hamper our ability in this area are an inability to listen and an inability to empathize with others.

Another thing which hampers church people in their pastoral ministry is a tendency, at times, to be too exacting, to carry the idea of perfection a bit too far. This kind of attitude often gives people the uncomfortable feeling that we are continually disappointed in them. If this happens, we cannot be truly present to the people we seek to serve.

Other attitudes that retard our ability to communicate include discourtesy, fault-finding, irritableness, and self-righteousness. We must continually strive to honestly assess our thoughts and attitudes to determine whether we really see others as truly our brothers and sisters in Christ. I am convinced that our ministry is vastly enhanced, that we are more therapeutic individuals, the closer we emulate the gentle Jesus.

In reaching out to others in time of need, it must never be our concern to add another person to the rolls of our churches. Our role is not to make the body of Christ more obese. Rather, we are called to exercise a therapeutic role, one which calls for deep commitment to and deep involvement in common human concerns. This involvement, at its core, can best be referred to as Christian presence — a true presence and availability to others which proceeds from the wholeness so freely given to us and which, as it is shared, becomes the vehicle through which effective healing flows. We have been touched, and it is our responsibility to touch others.